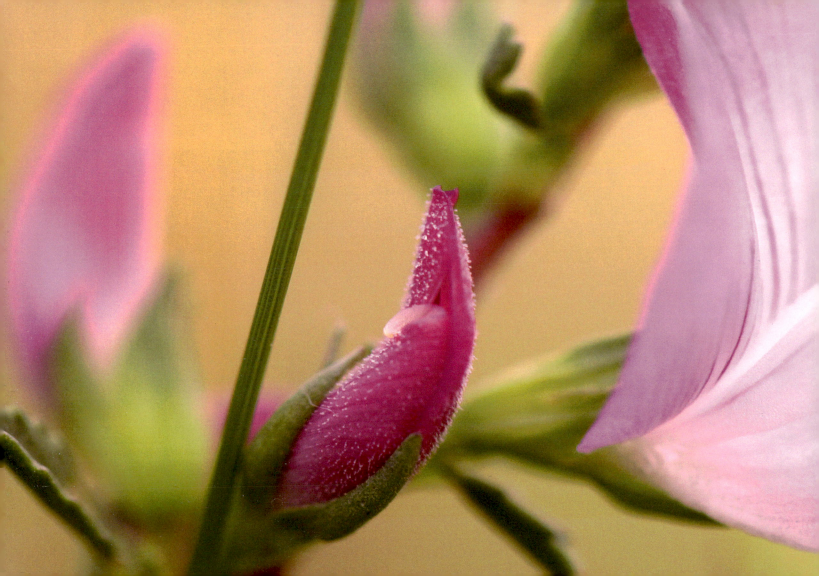

Table of Contents

Introduction — 1

Chapter 1 - Finding Joy — 3

Chapter 2 - Choosing the Better Part — 15

Chapter 3 - Drawing Inward — 25

Chapter 4 - Perseverance & Becoming Stronger — 35

Chapter 5 - Peace — 45

Chapter 6 - Forgiveness — 61

Chapter 7 - Accepting — 75

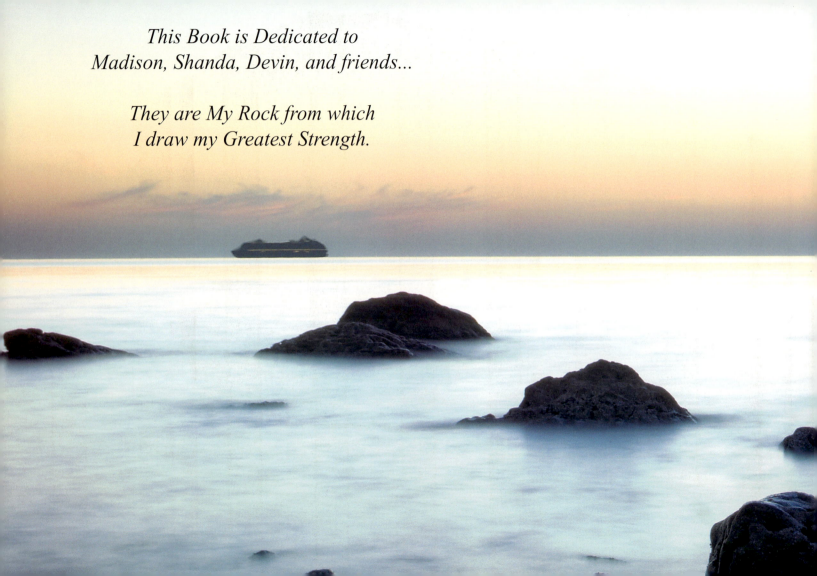

*This Book is Dedicated to
Madison, Shanda, Devin, and friends...*

*They are My Rock from which
I draw my Greatest Strength.*

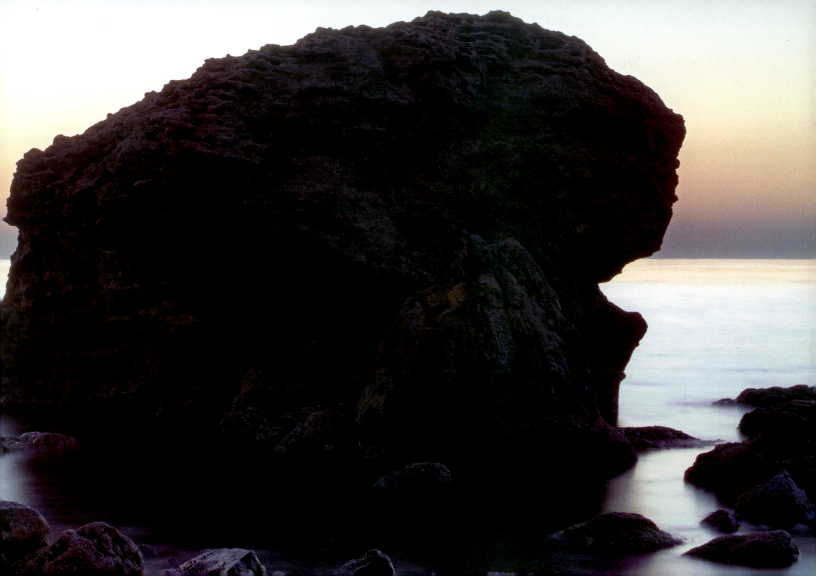

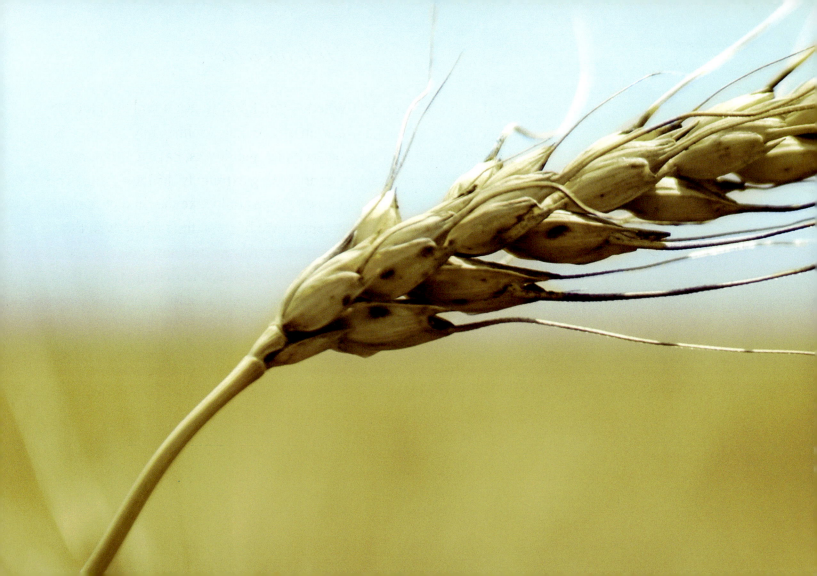

Introduction

YOU are extraordinary! Whether you know it or not you hold the key to your own emotional freedom. There may be times in your life when you might feel overwhelmed with up and downs, have a very long to-do list that never stops, or are facing extremely difficult times. This may leave you wondering how anyone could take the time to spend a few minutes on self improvement. We live in a time when "you time" might get pushed aside. Have you ever wondered how you can keep moving forward, partake of sweet happiness, and find the joy in the journey? There is a way to take a few minutes each day to look at yourself and see the true you. If you spend a little time each day and have recognized improvements.

As you press forward by using Young Living products you can push through unwanted emotions and start preparing and motivate yourself to understand emotional healing. Allow yourself some time each day to connect with you and your body by using these affirmations to find joy.

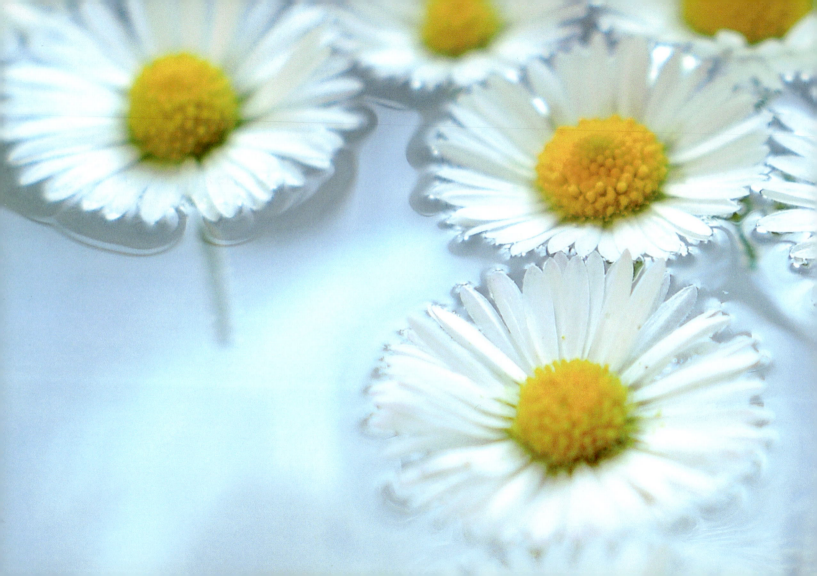

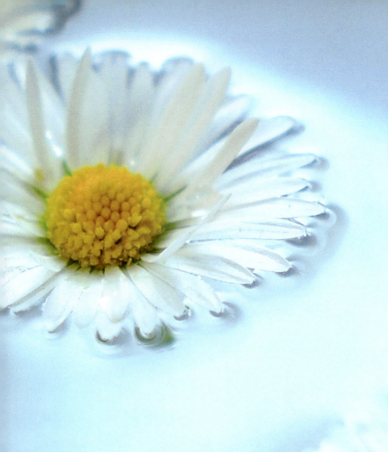

- Chapter 1 -
Finding Joy

Although life can have unexpected ups, downs, twists and turns, people can create the life and journey they desire. Create a firm foundation for yourself by focusing on love and security. You were born to have joy and to realize true happiness.

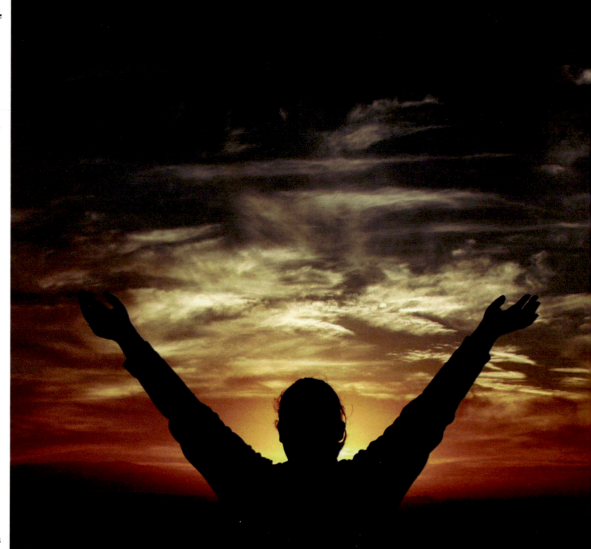

I apply *Joy* to my heart to create a firm foundation for the emotional freedom of my body, mind and soul. I approve of myself, take my power back and stand strong.

I love myself for who I am and what God/higher power gives me.

I allow my gifts, talents and others' experiences to teach me for my own growth.

I create a determination for joy and to love my life.

Refresh, Renew, Improve

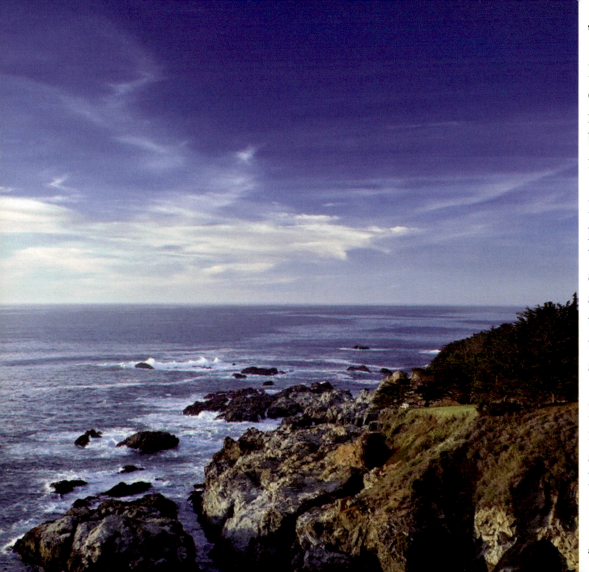

I rub *Harmony* on the sides of my body to protect myself and allow my body, mind and soul to feel joy.

I stand tall, seize my power and move forward with strength, conviction and unity of mind, body and soul. I allow myself to be in harmony with my true self and see myself as a joyful person.

I allow the good I have inside to come out and realize harmonic happiness.

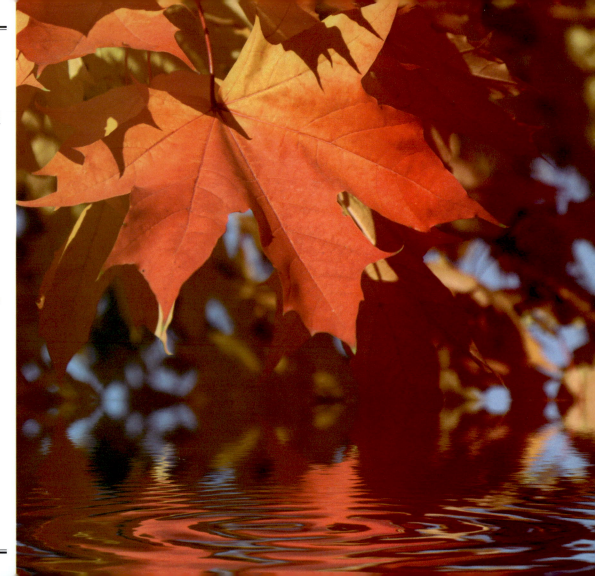

I hold *Highest Potential* over my shoulders and I support my thoughts and realize my great ability to create a joyful life.

I trust myself to reach my highest good.

I allow my body to start to relax by taking a deep breath and inhaling the source of deep peace.

I allow myself to feel a strength overcome my body, mind and soul to realize my highest potential.

Refresh, Renew, Improve

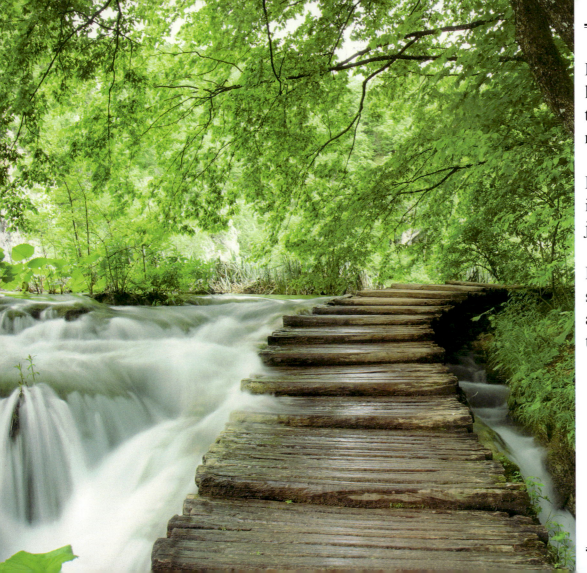

I apply *Juva Flex* to my liver and I allow the past to be in the past and allow myself to move forward.

I allow myself to progress in my life's journey with joyful determination.

I approve and create a space in myself where I allow bliss and peace all the time.

I apply *Cypress* to the body and I feel a freedom overcome my body as my energy flows freely.

I allow white light to flow through my body and fill me with joy.

I create only good in my body and seek the higher joy of life.

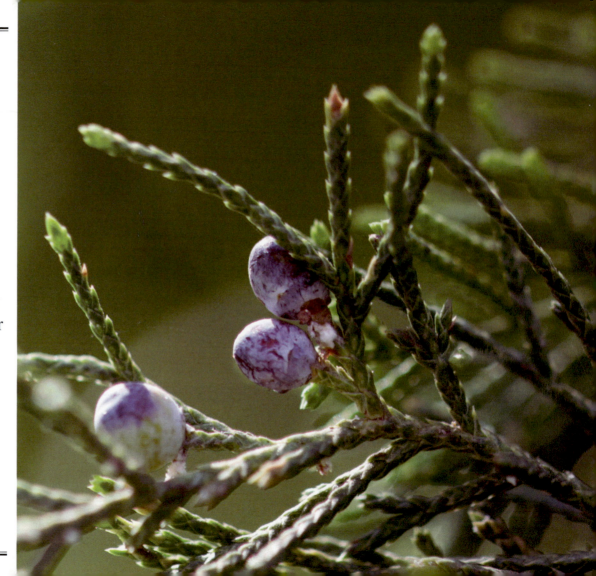

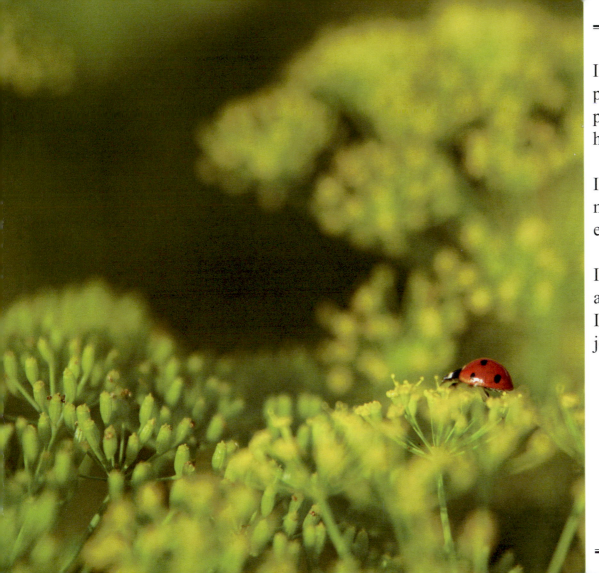

Refresh, Renew, Improve

I apply *Dill* to my Vitaflex points and I choose to be peaceful and realize harmonic joy.

I receive white light from my God/ higher power and enhance my self love.

I govern my body, mind and soul and create a life I choose to realize my joyful purpose.

I apply *Geranium* to my third eye and allow my body to freely see miracles that happen and create peace and joy for myself.

I allow myself to live in the here-and-now and encircle myself with love.

I feel my body, mind and soul with white light and realize ultimate joy.

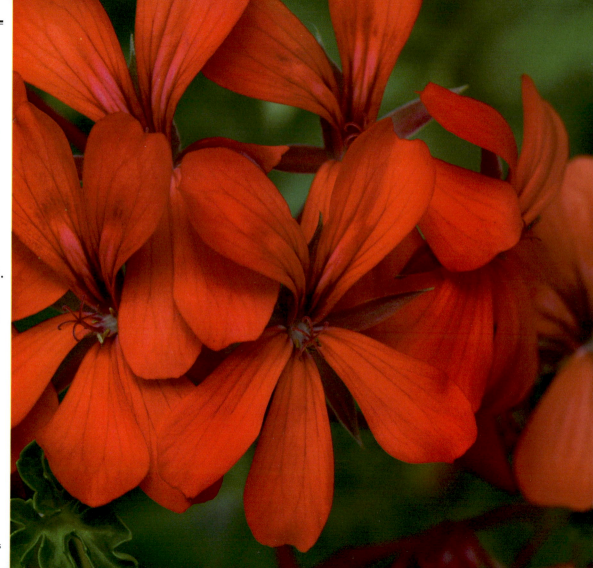

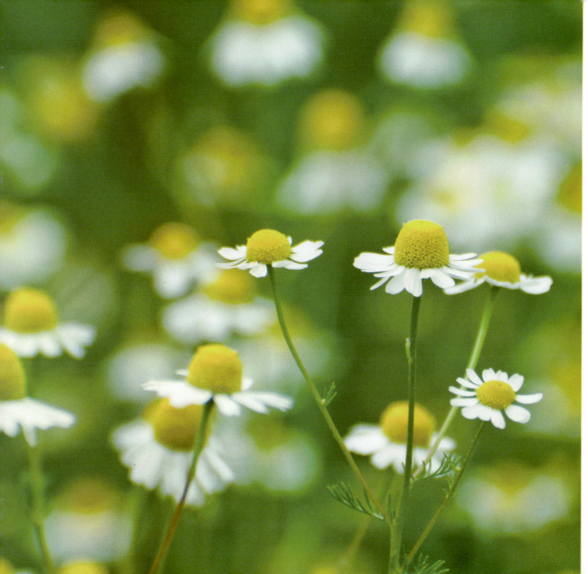

Refresh, Renew, Improve

I drink *German Chamomile* in almond milk and my soul sings with joy and happiness for all the strength I possess.

I am tolerant, kind and loving to all especially myself.

I always find opportunities and reasons to rejoice.

I hold *Ledum* in my hand over my liver and create faith and belief that with the help of my God/ higher power I can joyfully guide, direct and bless my life.

I govern myself to allow my body to be supported and I choose peace and joy.

I allow peace and harmony to surround me and I rejoice in creating a joyous and wonderful day.

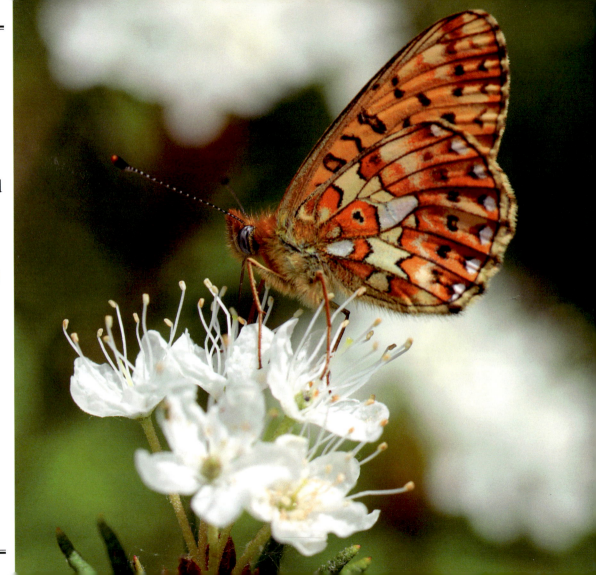

Refresh, Renew, Improve

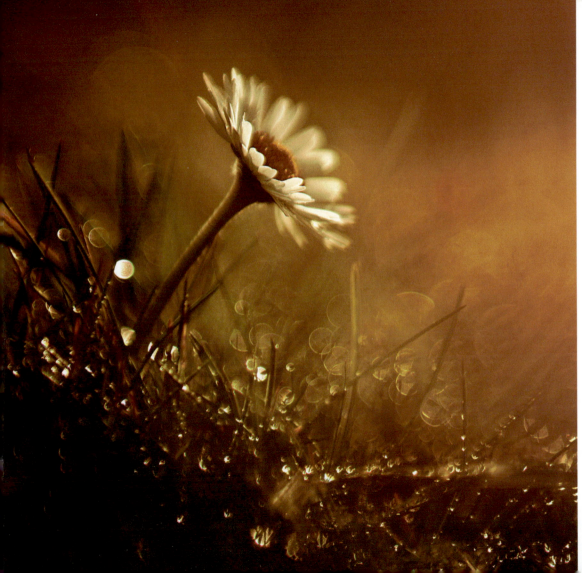

I rub *Peace & Calming* over the feet and I listen to and trust my inner-child.

On my journey in life I continually and easily proceed with calmness and serenity that fills my entire being with bliss and joy.

I allow myself a voice in joyfully realizing my emotional freedom.

I am in control of me and allow my love for myself to swiftly overcome me with joy.

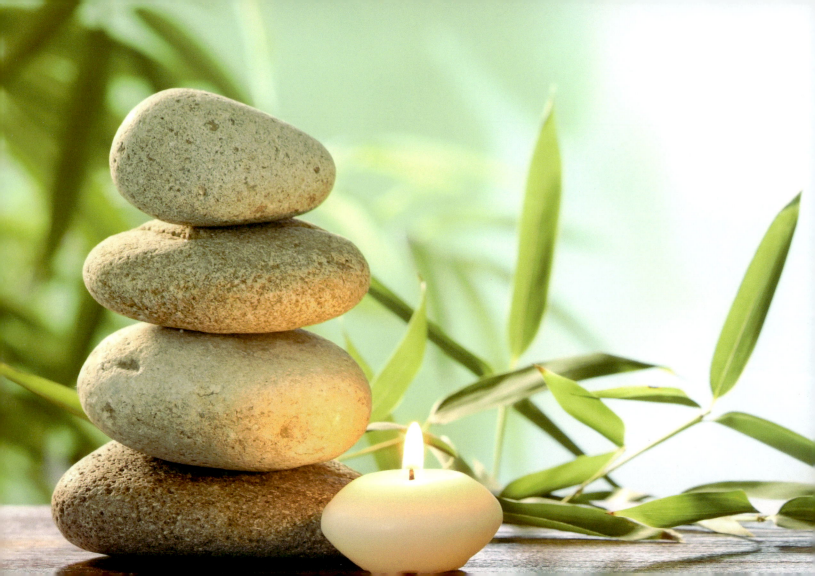

- Chapter 2 -
Choosing the Better Part

You possess the strength to become the person you are meant to be. It is possible to push yourself to a higher standard and realize your life's purpose with the assistance of your God/higher power. Improve and increase your white light and your ability to achieve all you were sent here to achieve.

Life's journey is about learning to grow and extending yourself a little more in order to expand and explode your vision. Your ability to press forward and reach worthwhile goals will expand. Keep yourself focused and express love to yourself each day.

I apply *Myrrh* over my head and allow it to balance my body, mind and soul to reach my ultimate level of mental and spiritual awareness.

I choose to hear only the good that I or people say to me.

I choose to build myself up and say only thoughtful and positive words about myself and others.

I am gentle with myself and others.

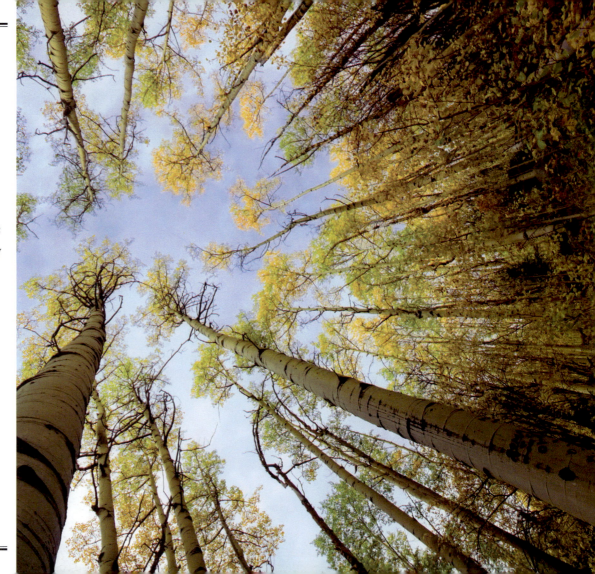

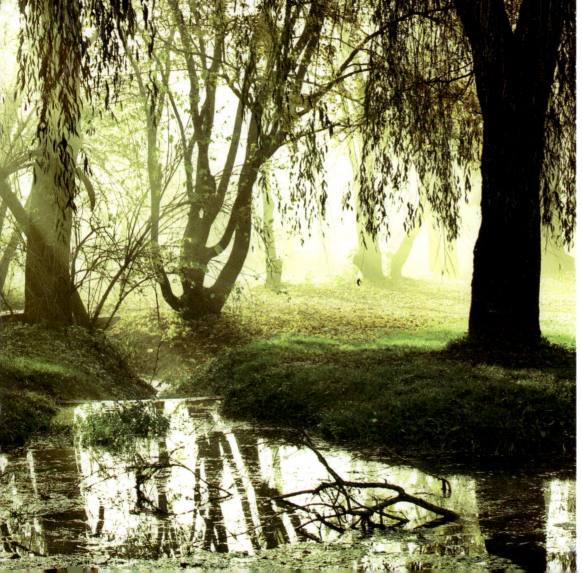

I apply *Melissa* to my sternum and I choose to allow it to protect and strengthen my body, mind and soul.

I leave my past experiences in the past and move forward with strength and conviction. I allow white light to fill my entire being.

I express peace to my body, mind and soul and create ultimate acceptance of myself.

I drip *Lime* oil over my head and feel harmony overtake my body.

I create clarity of vision for my future and realize I possess all the mental strength I need to realize my highest potential.

I allow the past to remain in the past and move forward with hope and obedience to my true self.

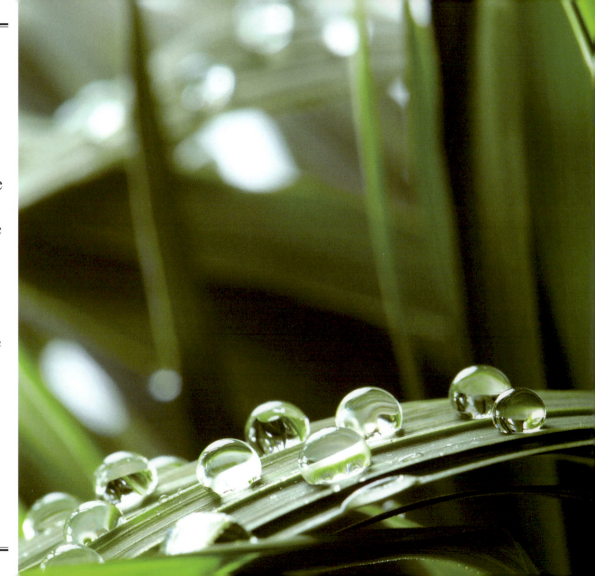

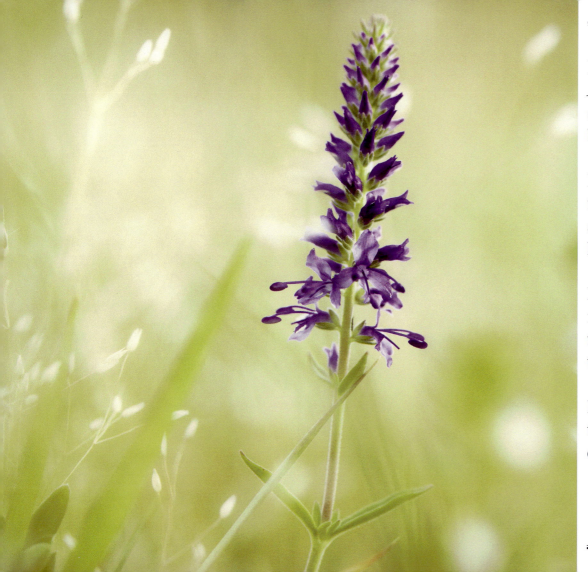

Refresh, Renew, Improve

I breathe in the power of *Lavender* and I encourage a peace to overcome my body, mind and soul.

I feel a grounding in the present to anchor all my hopes in the here-and-now.

I allow myself to trust me for the great good I give to myself, others and the world.

I choose to allow myself to stand strong with courage in the present.

I rub *Sensation* on my ankles and wrists, breathe it in and I develop and maintain a greater love for myself.

I choose confidence and experience grown from the past and allow my experiences to teach me what is necessary then move into the present.

I am safe, secure and forgiving to myself and others.

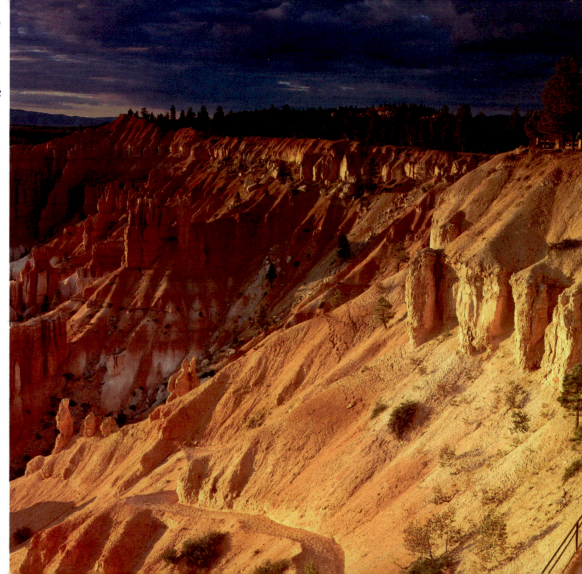

Refresh, Renew, Improve

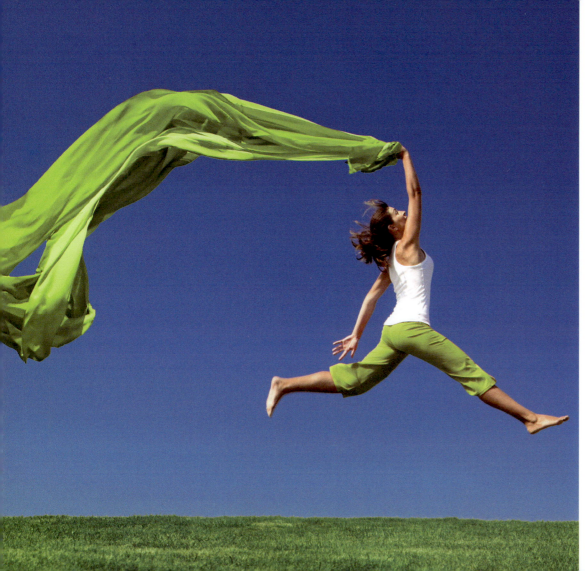

I apply *Surrender* to my forehead and I guide my body to release and surrender my path to my God/ higher power.

I choose to let my God/ higher power teach me how to be in control of my life and my potential.

I feel a new healing come over myself.

Refresh, Renew, Improve

I rub *Juniper* on my abdomen and I choose to set goals that immediately place me on a path to reach my highest potential.

I always forgive myself and allow myself to be cleared and purified from the past to create a renewed energy.

I connect with my inner-child and allow my body, mind and soul to constantly progress on a peaceful path.

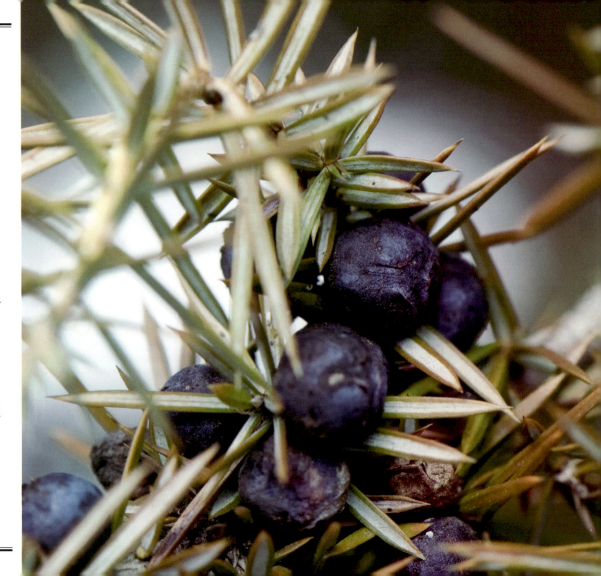

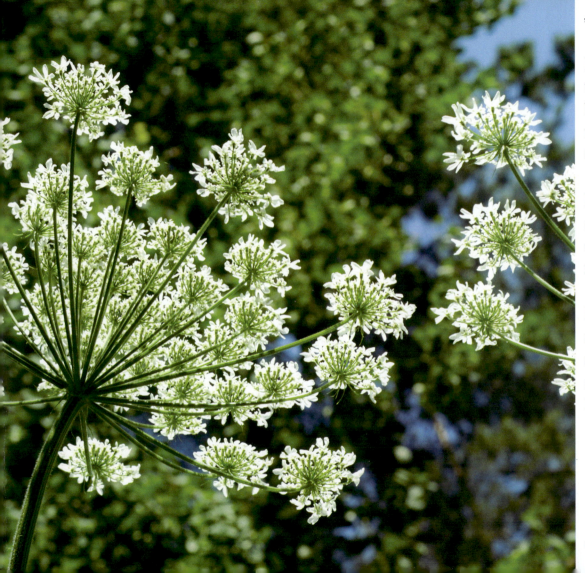

I apply *White Angelica* to my heart allowing my body to stand up for my true self as a creation of God/higher power.

I encourage myself to stand up to myself and others for the great good I really am.

I am progressing and I allow myself to be free and progress with ease and swiftness in realizing my highest potential.

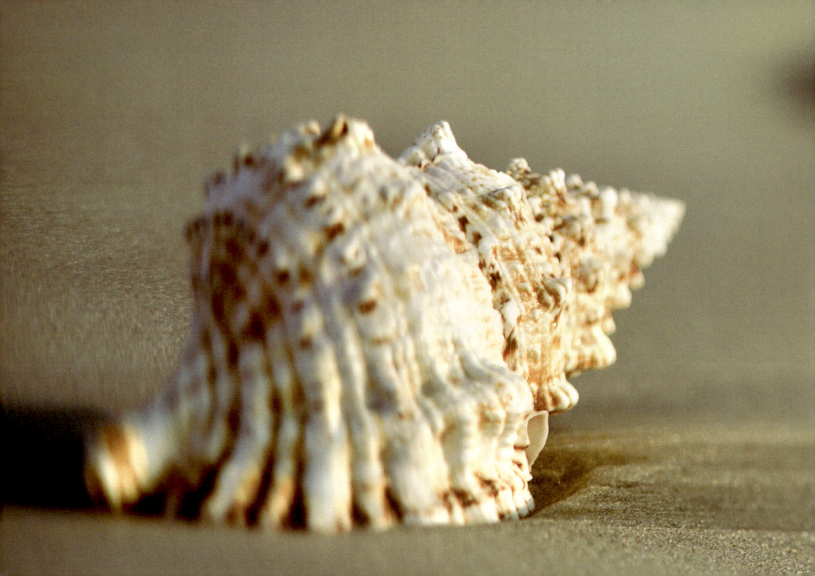

- Chapter 3 -
Drawing Inward

Allow yourself to see there is a foundation, then you can start to love yourself. Allow your body to feel protected and supported to see a strength inside you never noticed before. Permit yourself to look inward and learn to lean on your strength to grow. Feel a strength and energy allowing you to connect with your inner beauty and love who you are.

Feel a newfound love and create an inner strength to realize your highest potential. As you say the affirmations, pinpoint a few and work on them often. Then notice the change that starts to come over you. Allow a new light to shine from within your soul and open up your mind to live to your fullest and love yourself.

I rub *Valor* to the bottom of my feet and I participate in memorable experiences that allow me to draw inward to support and protect me.

I choose to feel an inward peace full of safety, protection and courage.

I allow my life to be protected and I speak up for myself in loving ways.

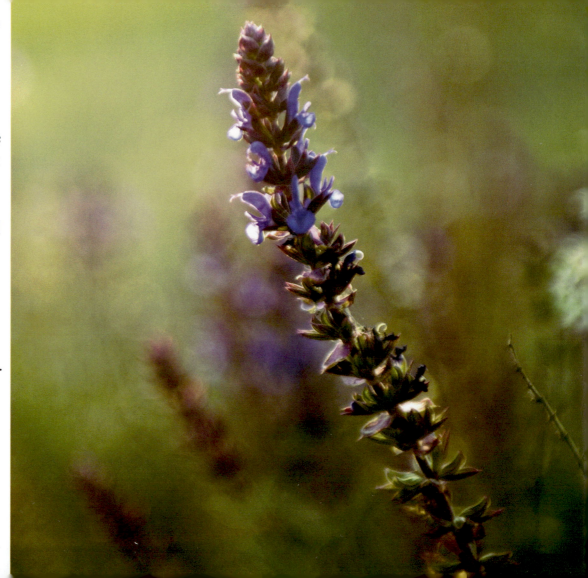

Refresh, Renew, Improve

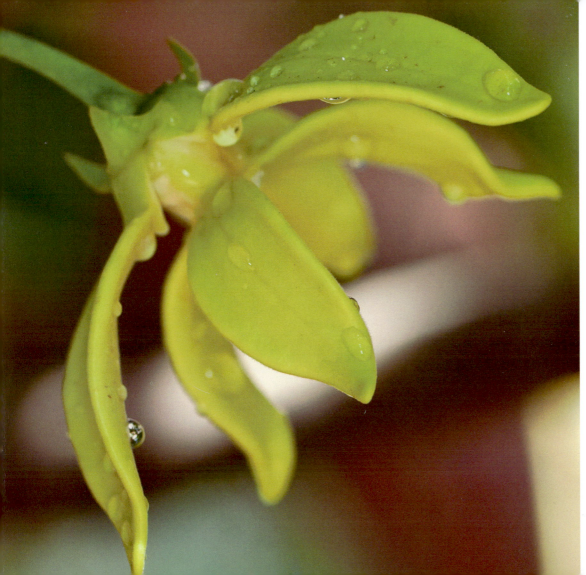

I put it *Ylang Ylang* over my bed at night, indulge in the beautiful smell and live a balanced life.

I feel a great love for myself generating from deep inside my being.

I plan and bring a feeling of self-love for myself and my mate.

I rub a few drops of *Spikenard* on my feet at night and guide my body, mind and soul to a peaceful and safe space.

I balance and represent my inner-self to bring my soul to a higher place.

I feel at peace and at one with my inner-self and my God/higher power.

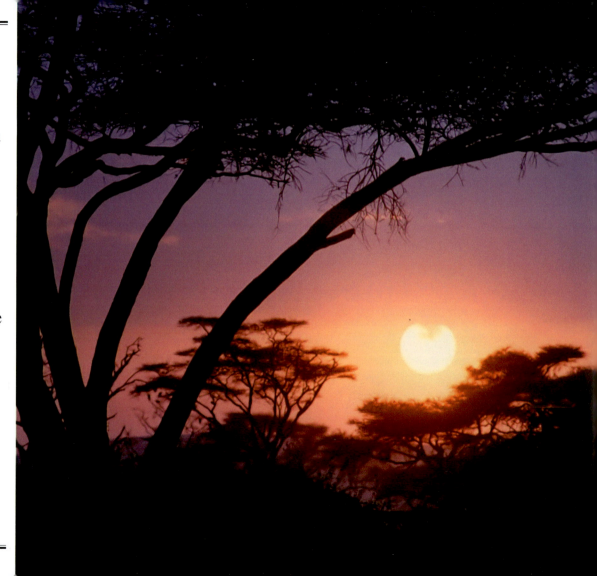

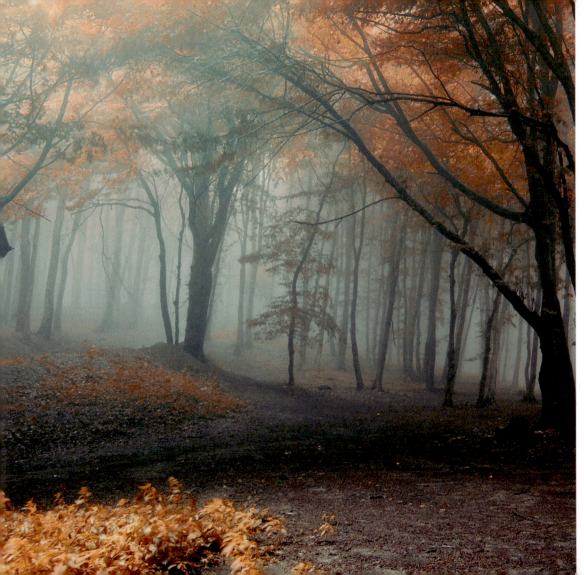

Refresh, Renew, Improve

I rub *Sandalwood* in my hands and I connect with my inner-self, allowing my full power to radiate outward and shine.

I only allow positive programming to take over my body, mind and soul.

I organize a high path for me to follow and generate greatness within me to realize my highest potential.

I apply *Frankincense* to my feet and I allow the full power to fill my whole body, mind and soul, then move forward with joy.

I feel a divine protection and white light overcome my body, mind and soul to strengthen me inwardly.

I am totally safe in the space I created and only allow good to enter.

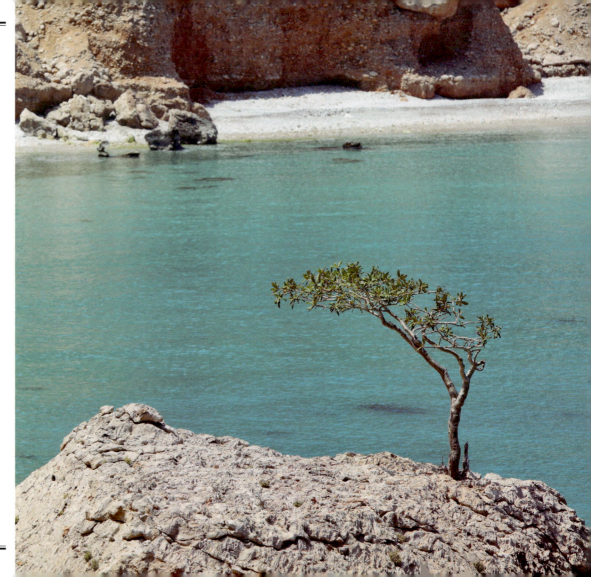

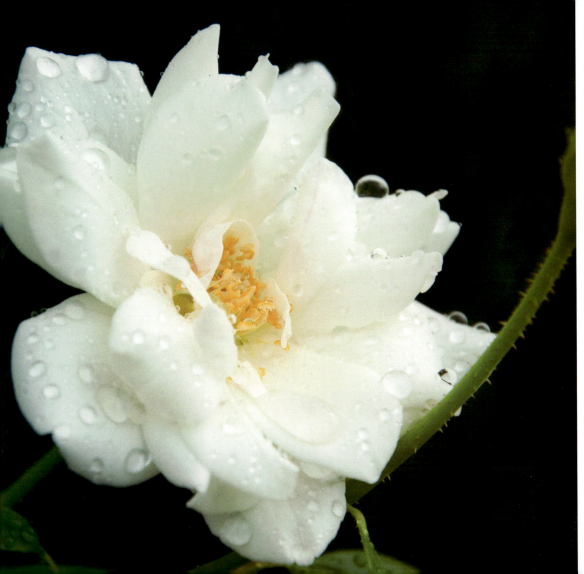

Refresh, Renew, Improve

I rub *Rose* over my face, allow it to penetrate my body and strengthen me and I see the beauty I am from the inside out.

I guide myself to a better path and program my mind to see the great purpose for me.

I allow my inner-child to be strong and play a big part in moving me forward.

I place *Orange* over my heart and I continually tell myself I am strong.

I feel an inward peace guide and direct me in realizing my life's purpose.

I am strong from deep within and progress forward with ease in realizing my highest potential.

I allow joy to perpetuate from inside of me and overcome my body, mind and soul.

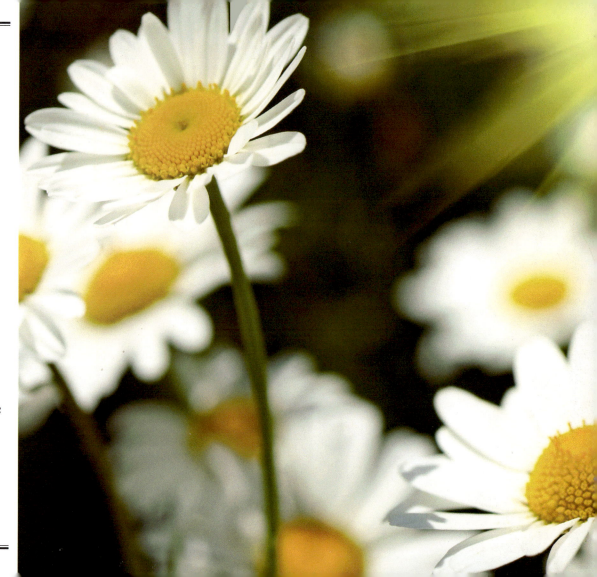

Refresh, Renew, Improve

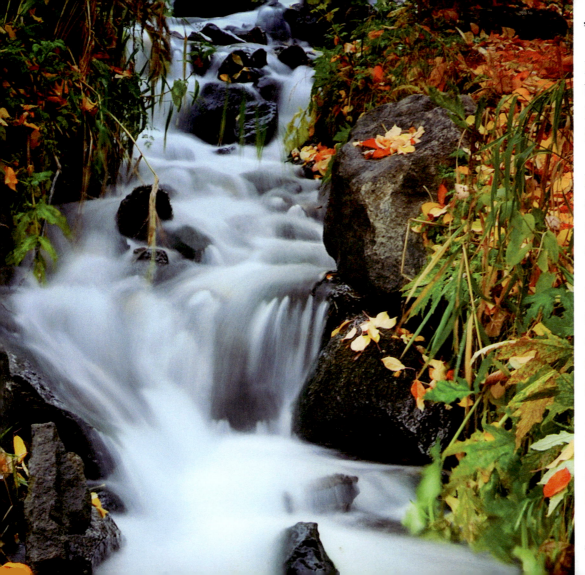

I add *Myrtle* to my healthy beverage; drink it in and I generate a strong inner-peace.

Beginning within my core-self I live a stronger, productive and abundant life.

I write a plan for myself that will take me on an excellent quest to realize my highest potential and a great life.

I encourage and facilitate a stronger inner-self to enrich and heighten my body, mind and soul.

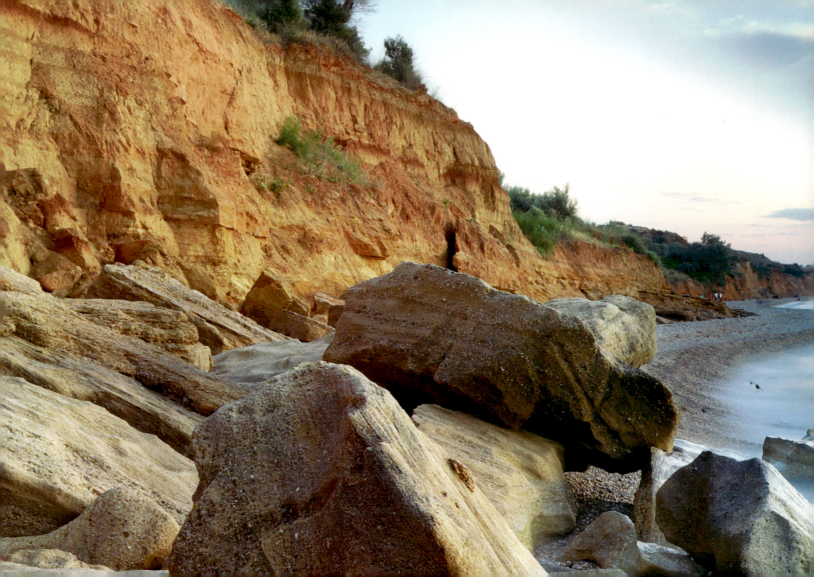

Chapter 4
Perseverance & Becoming Stronger

Allow essential oils to be an integrated part of your life and permit yourself to discover the joy in persevering with a strong purpose. This is the time in your life to become strong and fully utilize your light. It is time to find strength and allow your body, mind and soul to be strong and persevere in realizing your highest potential.

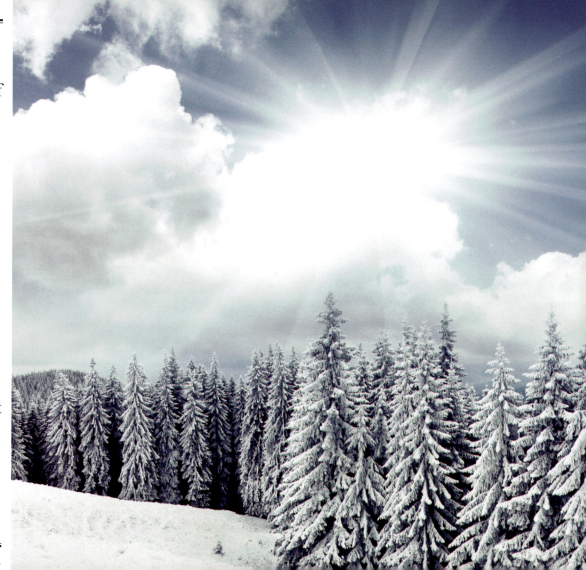

I place *Hope* to the rim of my ears and breath in the joy of choosing to move forward with ease and great perseverance.

I focus on an inner-peace that empowers my innate ability to easily and persistently continue on the road to my highest potential.

I possess the faith and hope necessary to present a strong life. The light of my God/ higher power gives me the strength on my quest to realize my highest potential.

Refresh, Renew, Improve

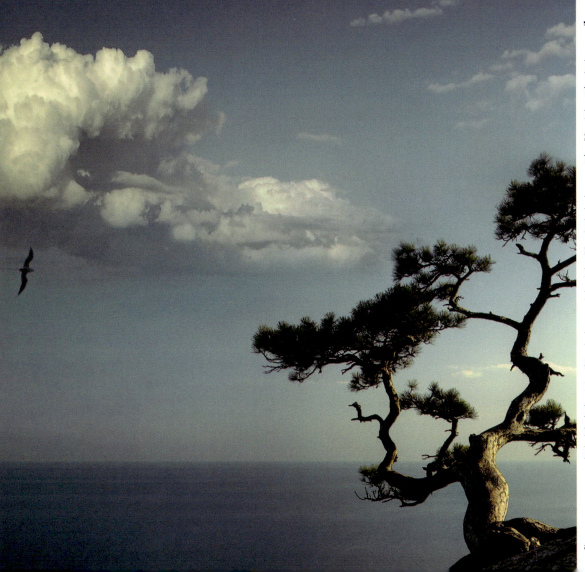

I rub *Humility* over my temples and hold for a few seconds, and feel the soothing strength it gives to my mind and soul.

I operate at the highest level of motivation and strength to progress forward with emotional freedom.

In great humility I accept the white light from my God/ higher power to easily guide me on my path to my highest potential.

I inhale *Live With Passion* deep into my inner-being and allow my body, mind and soul to feel great confidence and exceptional courage.

I allow myself to become powerful on my journey to reach my highest potential.

My life is the greatest gift from my God/higher power that I possess and I am a worthy steward of life and my life's purpose.

I choose to use my life's passion to reach my highest potential for the greater good of myself and humankind.

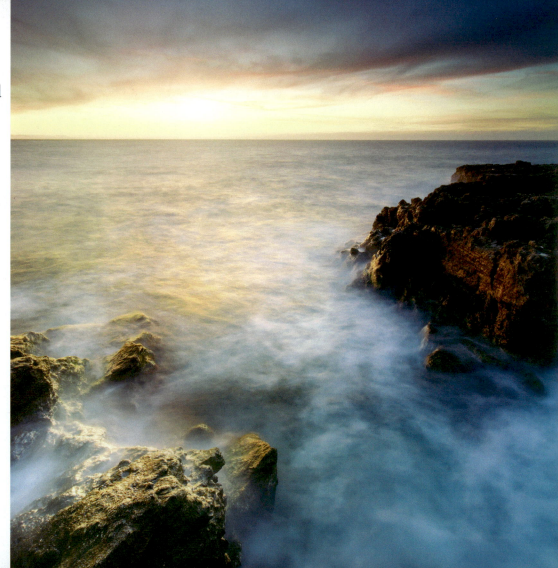

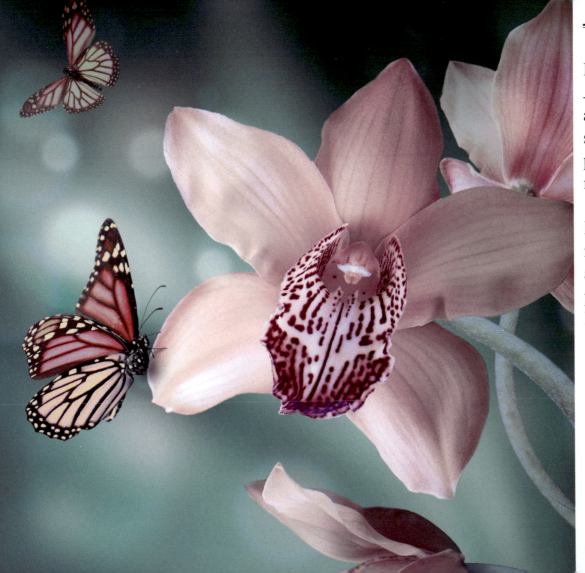

Refresh, Renew, Improve

I place *Magnify Your Purpose* on my shoulders and focus on my inherent strength to persistently progress forward to realize my highest potential.

I magnify and enhance my ability to persevere and move forward to progressively realize my life's purpose.

I wear *Motivation* on my wrist and I am persistently achieving my goals set this year.

I express love and acceptance to my body and allow my body to increase my strength.

I am ambitious and choose to accomplish my life's mission and purpose.

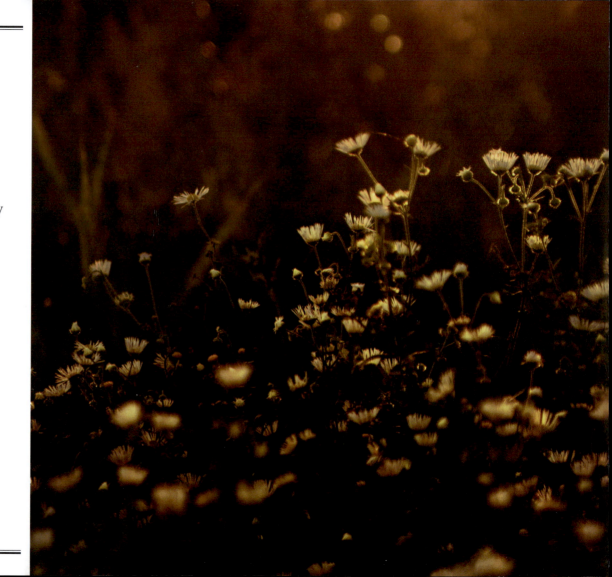

Refresh, Renew, Improve

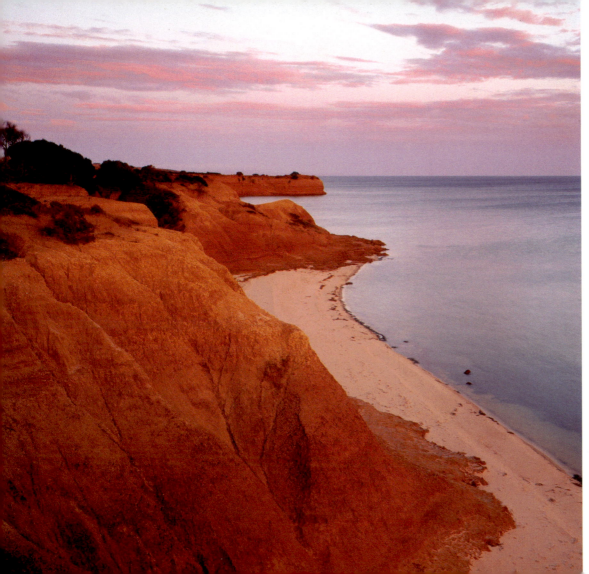

I rub *En-R-Gee* on my feet and tell myself I am making my life energetic and powerful.

I am extremely alive and feel a zest for living my life to the fullest and my highest potential.

I allow myself to be uplifted by my God/higher power and enjoy my life now.

I hold *Awaken* in my hand and over my sternum and I empower myself to visualize the road that is necessary to realize my highest potential.

I choose to empower myself to be emotionally free and allow my body, mind and soul to persevere and awaken to a higher potential.

I awaken to the talents that I have been given and allow my self to move forward with strength and ease.

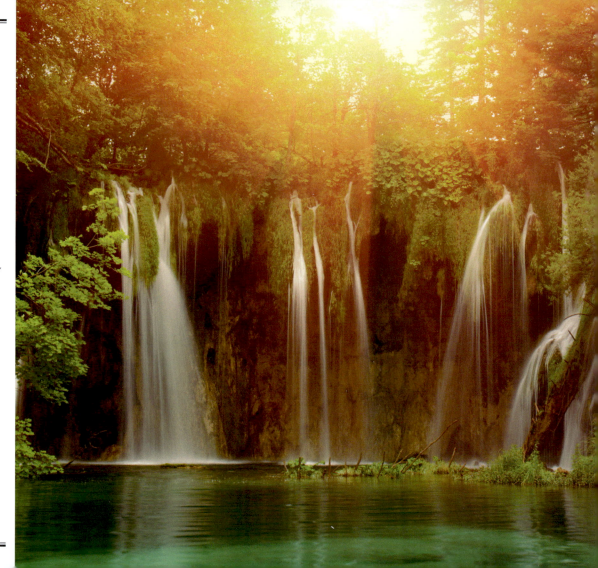

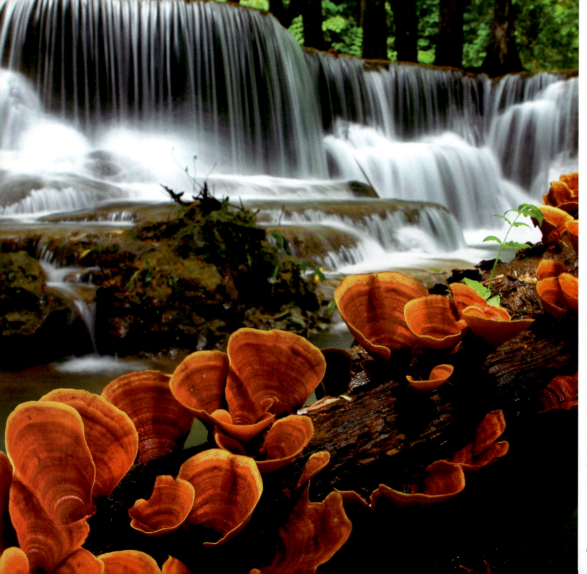

Refresh, Renew, Improve

I rub *Acceptance* in my hands and thank the past for the lessons I learned then move forward loving my new and worthwhile life.

I feel a great acceptance and love for the strength my God/higher power endowed me with to realize my highest potential.

I create a space of acceptance for my innate ability and power to persevere and increase my inner strength.

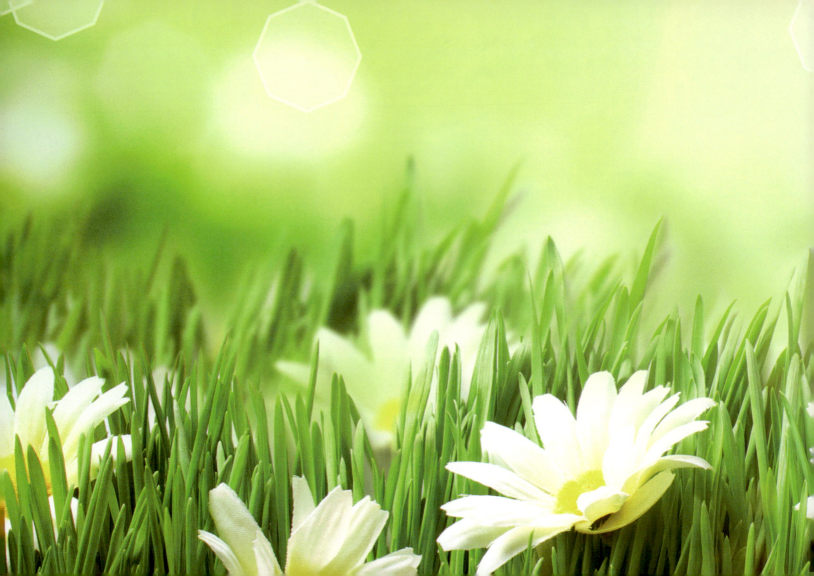

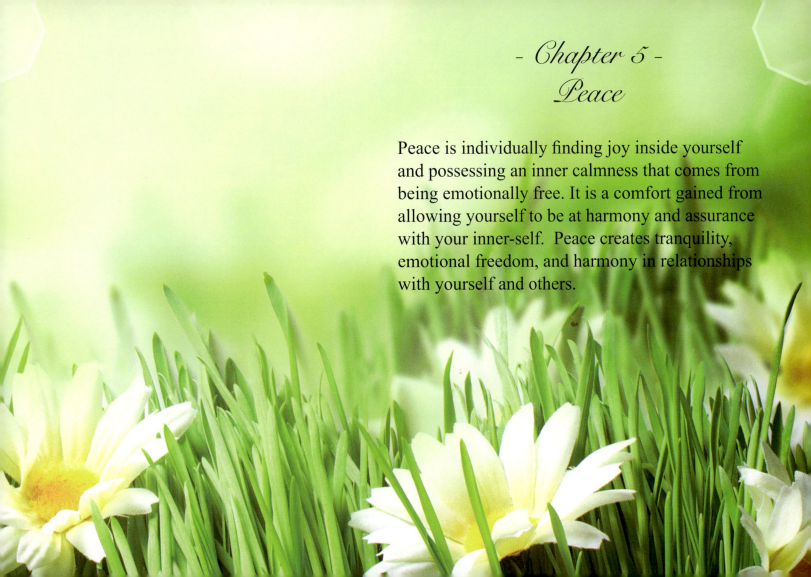

- Chapter 5 -
Peace

Peace is individually finding joy inside yourself and possessing an inner calmness that comes from being emotionally free. It is a comfort gained from allowing yourself to be at harmony and assurance with your inner-self. Peace creates tranquility, emotional freedom, and harmony in relationships with yourself and others.

I joyfully diffuse *Christmas Spirit* and I center my life in increased healing and wellness of body, mind and soul.

I encourage a positive outlook and allow myself to learn and grow from all my life's experiences.

I accept the strength given me by my God/higher power to create a peaceful and abundant life.

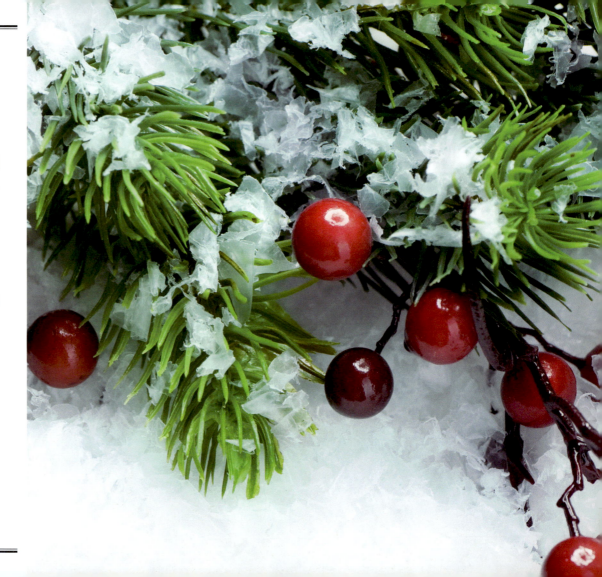

Refresh, Renew, Improve

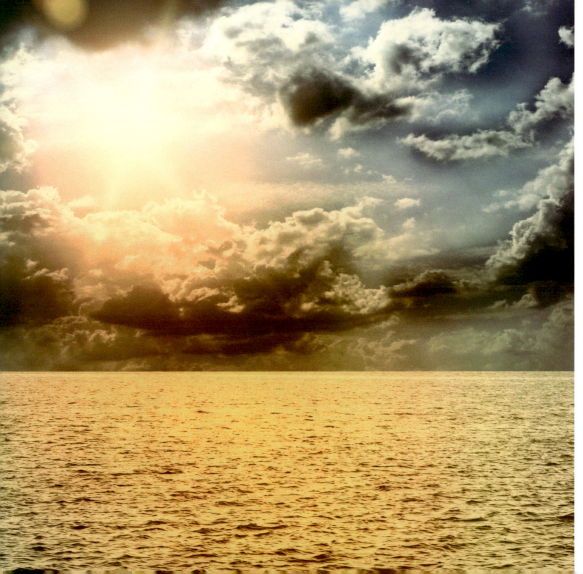

I apply *Believe* over my heart and I allow an inner peace to surround my body, mind and soul.

I possess faith, hope and courage that I can easily obtain inner peace and strength of body, mind and soul.

I am obedient to my true self and accept tranquility in utilizing white light to abundantly guide me in life's journey to reach my highest potential.

I hold fast to positive emotions.

I put *Awaken* on my hand; inhale it and I feel miracles happen in my body.

I allow myself to activate inner-peace and happiness in my body, mind and soul.

I kindle my inner desire for peace and awareness to grant myself the ability to reach my highest potential.

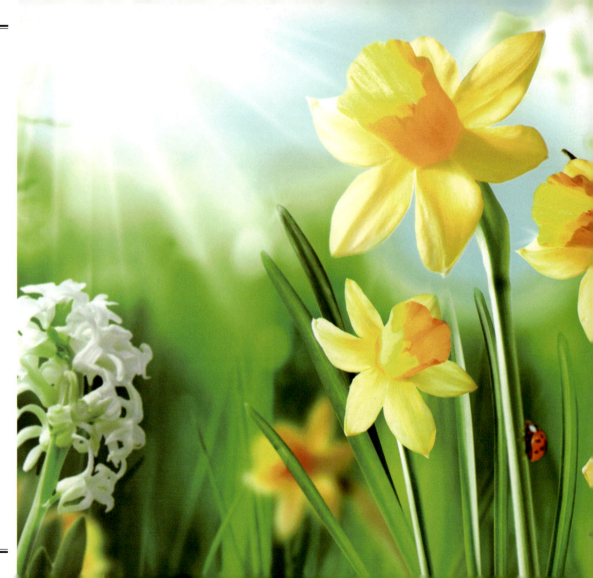

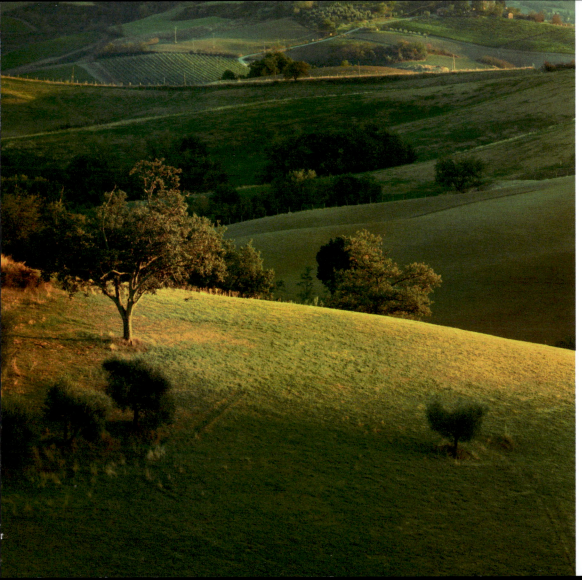

Refresh, Renew, Improve

I inhale *Sacred Mountain* and choose to find solace in my inner-self.

I choose to handle each situation separately, clearly and peacefully with individualized gentleness and love.

As I look for tranquility and I realize that peace may come in many diverse ways.

I realize and accept that I can possess peace and harmony in my life flowing from my God/higher power.

I inhale the beautiful smell of *Joy* and let its loving fragrance fill my whole body, mind and soul creating an exquisite inner-tranquility.

I let joy and solace come into the center of my being and encompass my body, mind and soul.

I grant myself to move ahead of the past and love myself for who I really am now.

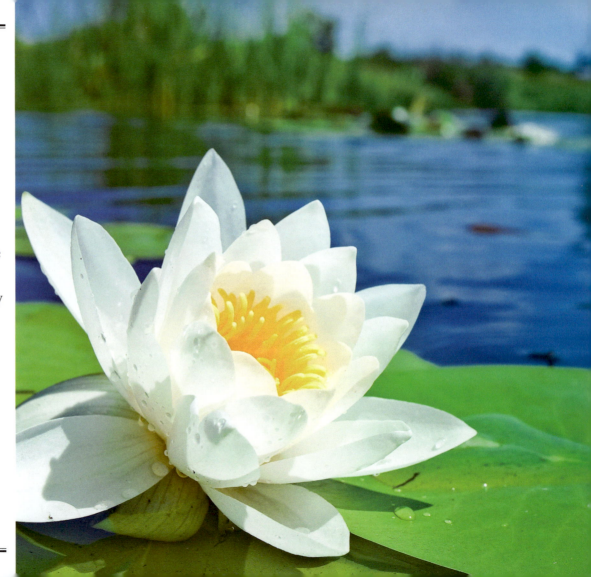

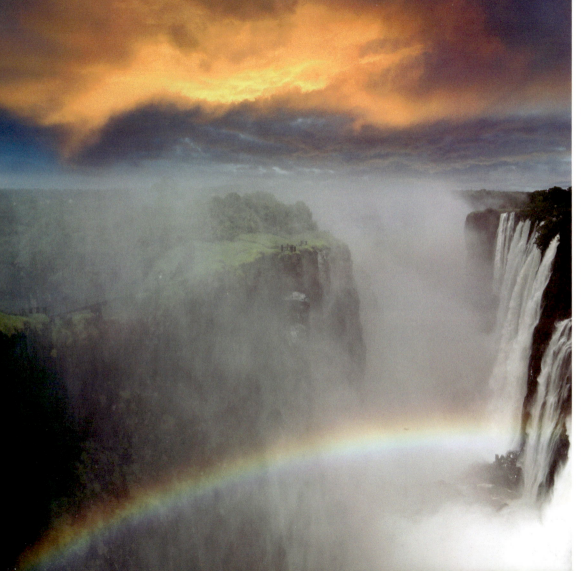

Refresh, Renew, Improve

I diffuse the oil of *Inspiration* and let go of the fear, allowing peace to enter my body, mind and soul as I freely breathe the power of spiritual awareness and calmness.

I allow myself to visualize peace encircling my body, mind and soul more abundantly than ever before.

I accept white light into my entire being and allow peace and harmony to engulf my body, mind and soul.

I rub *Into the Future* between my eyebrows and let the past remain in the past while moving forward with tranquility, excitement and joy in realizing a new future.

I allow past experiences to stay in the past and feel a harmony and peace of moving forward in allowing myself to approve of me.

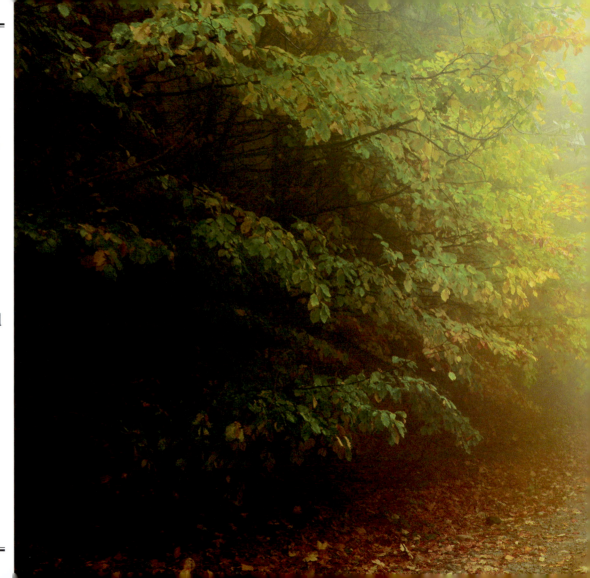

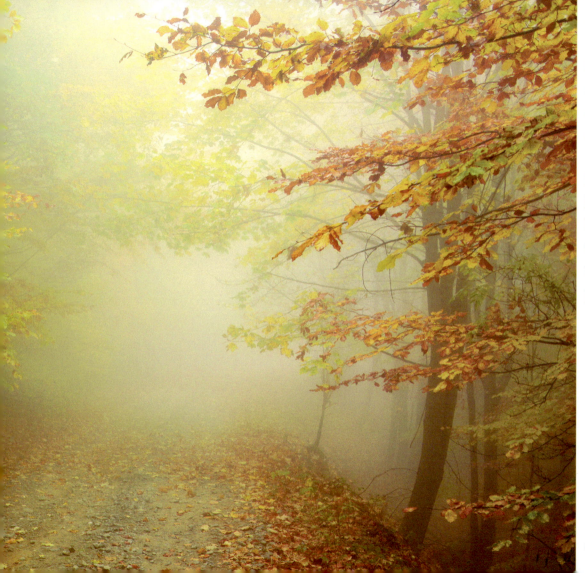

Refresh, Renew, Improve

I experience a hopeful and bright future full of harmony, tranquility, abundance and love.

I accept and allow harmonic positive feed back from my inner-self to guide my life's quest to reach my highest potential.

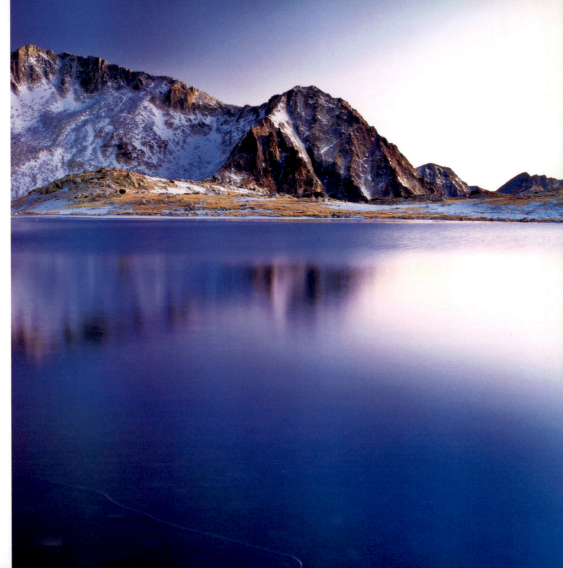

I apply *Peace and Calming* to my bed then allow myself to feel calm and accept peace into my life now.

I am able to live in peace and harmony with myself and my world.

I feel harmonic white light encircle my body, mind and soul to guide and direct me on my life's journey to realize my highest potential.

I realize my personal power creates a new inner-peace that fills my body, mind and soul with abundant harmony.

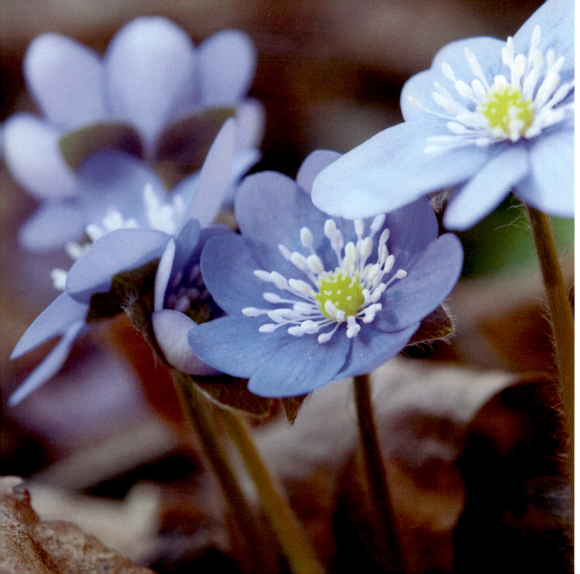

Refresh, Renew, Improve

I rub *Present Time* over my throat and allow myself to be in the moment and stay in control of my life in the here-and-now.

I express and observe a peace inside myself now and see a bright future to realize my life's purpose.

I permit myself to create a peaceful here-and-now to perceive a bright future.

I apply *Relieve It* to areas of deep tissue pain and I feel safe inside myself within the peacefulness I create for my body, mind and soul.

I create a space in my body to abundantly receive and to give.

My life's structure is strong enough to create peace for my body, mind and soul.

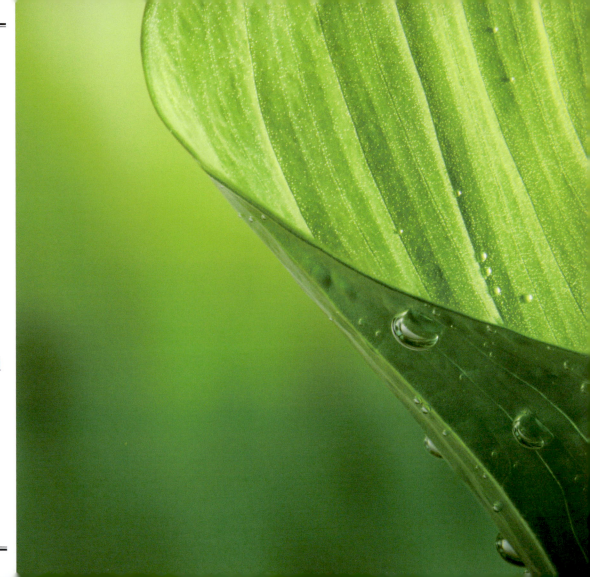

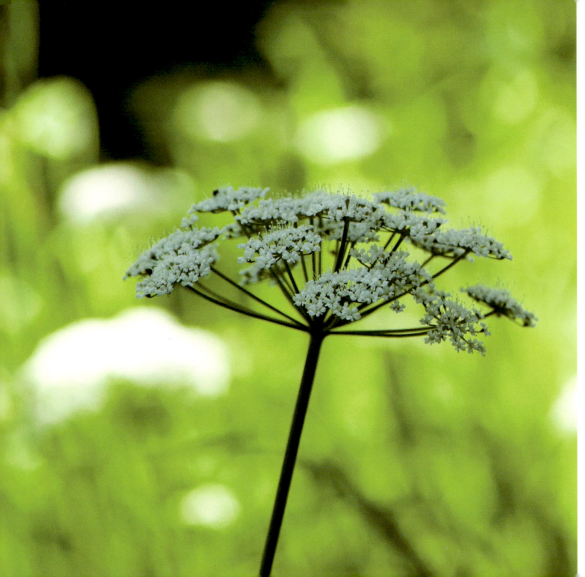

Refresh, Renew, Improve

I apply *White Angelica* to my shoulders and allow myself to be protected at the highest level.

I provide a safe space of harmony and love where I feel grounded and protected on my journey to reach my highest potential.

I organize and release any negative thought that might stop me from processing the light.

Refresh, Renew, Improve

I apply *Citrus Fresh* to the rim of my ears and let the oil improve and balance my system.

I am at peace with my past and free to move forward with renewed invigoration.

I am good enough to move forward and find an inner peace that supports my life.

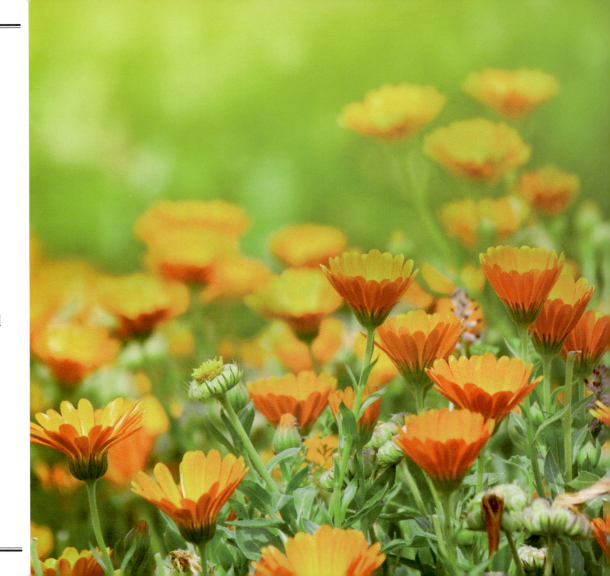

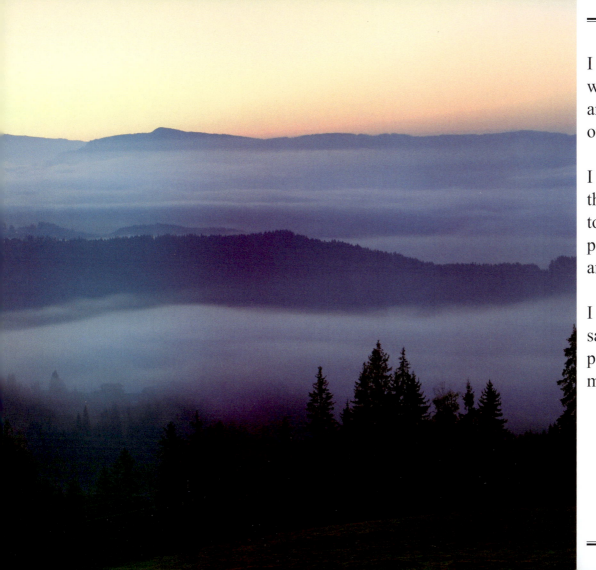

Refresh, Renew, Improve

I wear *Tranquil* on my wrist and feel a gentleness and a positive attitude overcome me.

I believe in me and the greatness I possess to realize my highest potential with calmness and serenity.

I allow myself to be safe, protected and at peace with myself and my world.

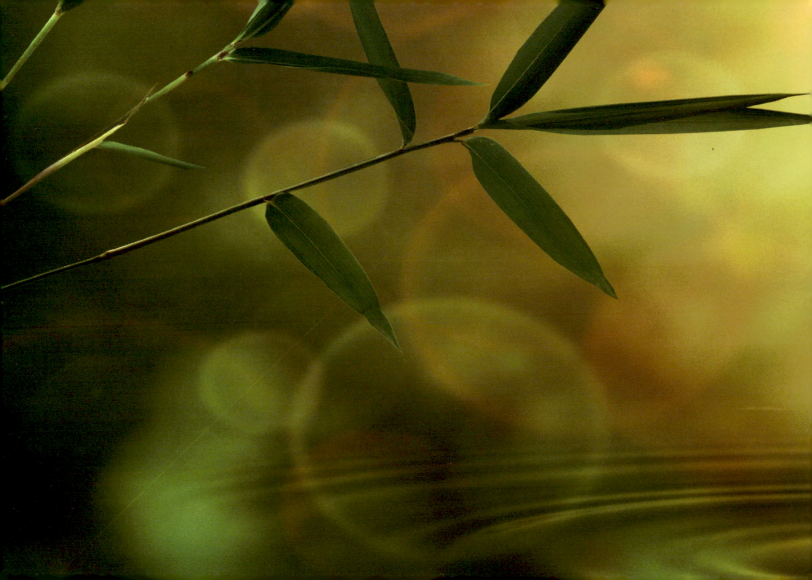

- Chapter 6 -
Forgiveness

Sometimes in life people may attempt to persuade you to detour from your life's journey. These roadblocks do not have to stop your progress to reach your highest potential. As you go beyond the speed bumps of life, you may find it necessary to forgive others and yourself which is necessary in order to fully progress. The ability to forgive can easily be enhanced by using essential oils and affirmations.

I drop *Valor* on my back and allow any feelings of courage and love to fill my body, mind and spirit.

I express love to my body and confidence to forgive myself and others.

I choose to forgive and create the courage to move forward and allow myself to love me.

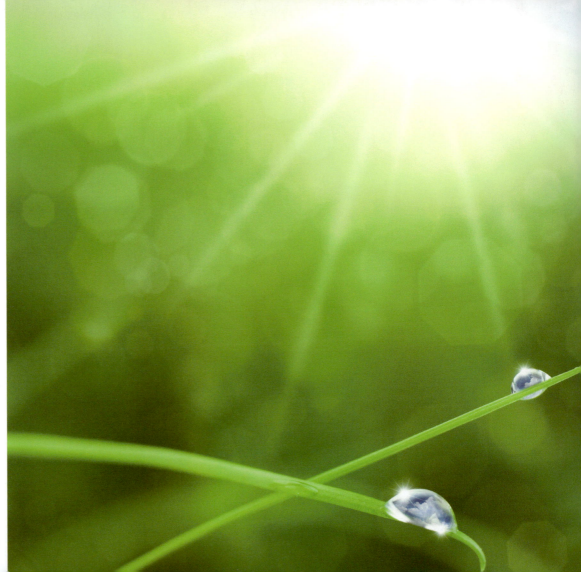

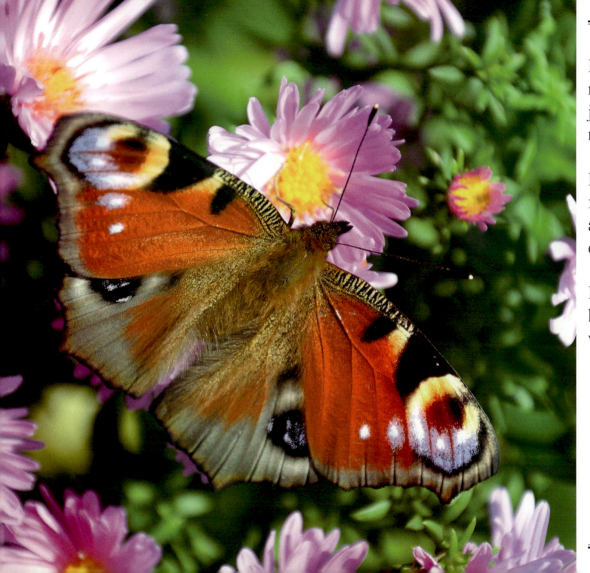

Refresh, Renew, Improve

I place *Forgiveness* over my heart and feel comfort, joy and love fill my body, mind and soul.

I possess courage to forgive myself and others and I move forward with confidence and ease.

I allow myself to feel and handle all my experiences with love and joy.

I place *Inner Child* on my navel and I begin to reconnect with my true core self.

I am strong and I choose to fill my body, mind and soul with courage and peace.

I continually realize the greatness within me to progress and move forward with strength and power.

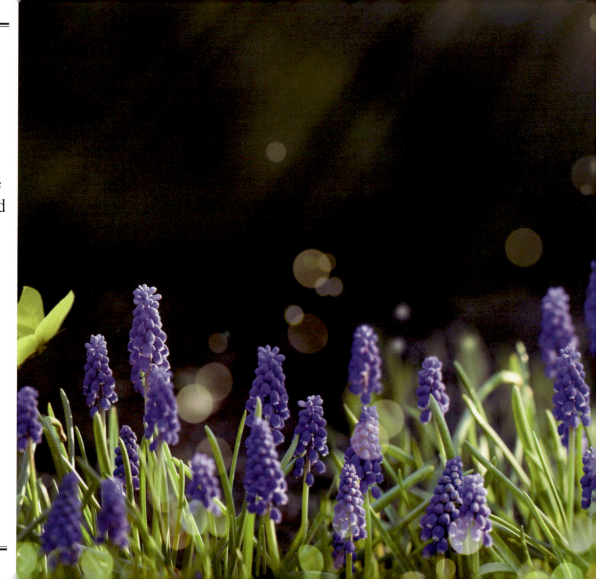

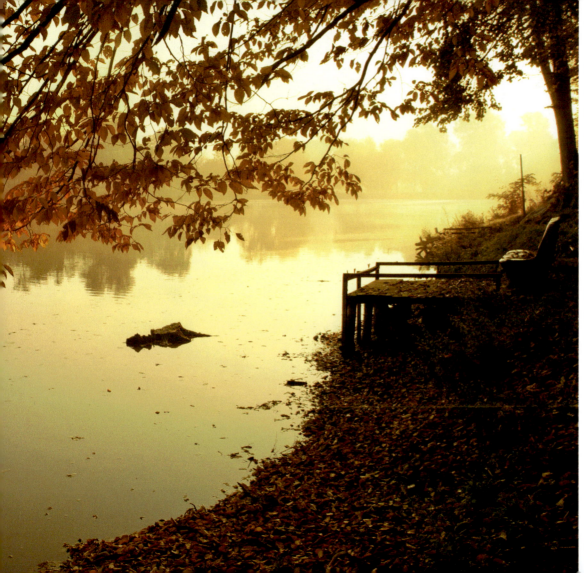

Refresh, Renew, Improve

I rub *Harmony* up and down the outside of my legs and I create unity with my true inner-self.

I am forgiving of myself and others and I create a greater harmony within my body, mind and soul.

I create wholeness to facilitate compassion for others and myself.

I hold *Release* over my liver and I let go of the pain and hurt that no longer serves me.

I freely feel love toward myself and others.

I offer my body light and love and choose to show empathy to let my power shine.

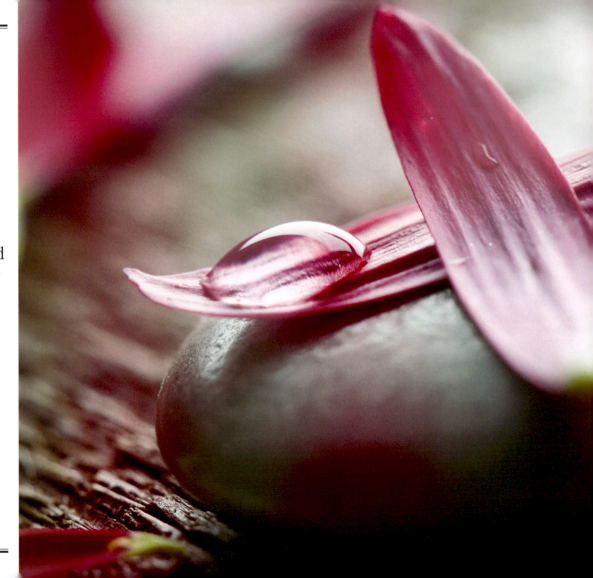

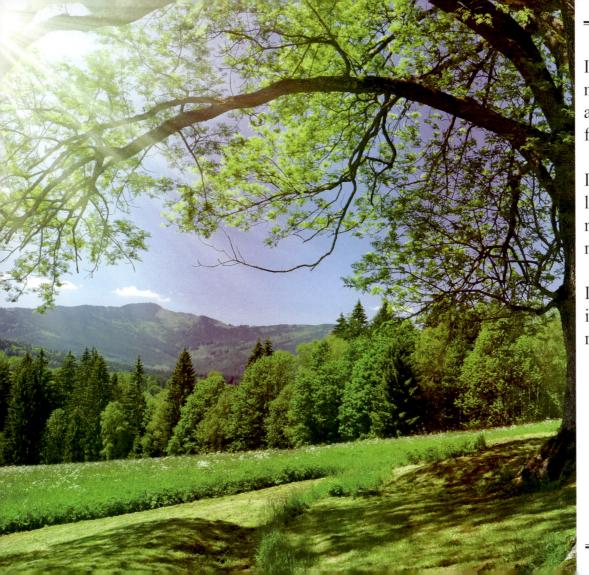

Refresh, Renew, Improve

I place *Trauma Life* over my lower back and allow myself to progress forward without difficulty.

I am surrounded with the light of love that increases my appreciation for myself and others.

I accept the process to incorporate safety in my healing.

I join my hands together and hold *Sara* over my navel and I let security enter my being.

I am protected and feel peace and security that I can achieve my highest good.

I treat others with loving respect and charity.

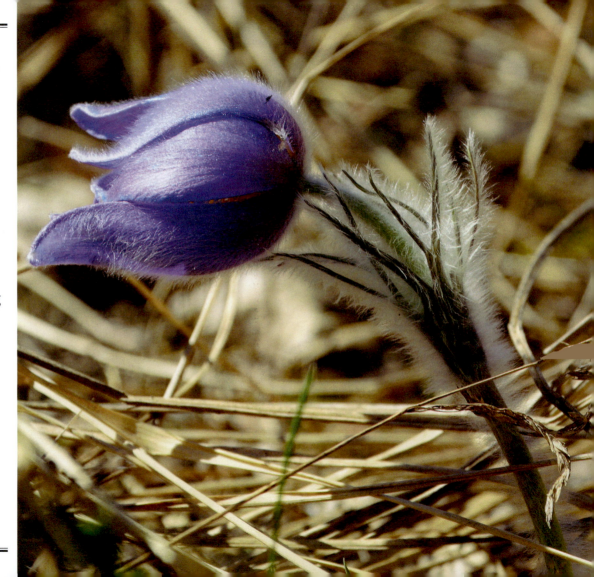

Refresh, Renew, Improve

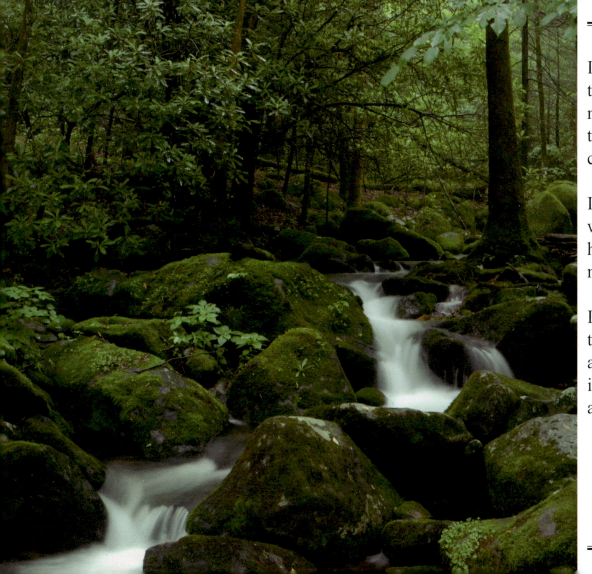

I drip *Surrender* over the top of my head and I allow my God/higher power to assist me in creating compassion for others.

I leave my emotional well-being to my God/higher power to enhance my life now.

I choose to understand the events in my life and allow benevolence to enter into my life with calmness and see myself safe.

I drip (*Three Wise Men*) on the top of the head and I allow myself to make wise decisions in improving my emotions.

I possess the absolute wisdom to make the best choices in forgiving and improving myself.

I allow myself to be in the moment and create a positive attitude.

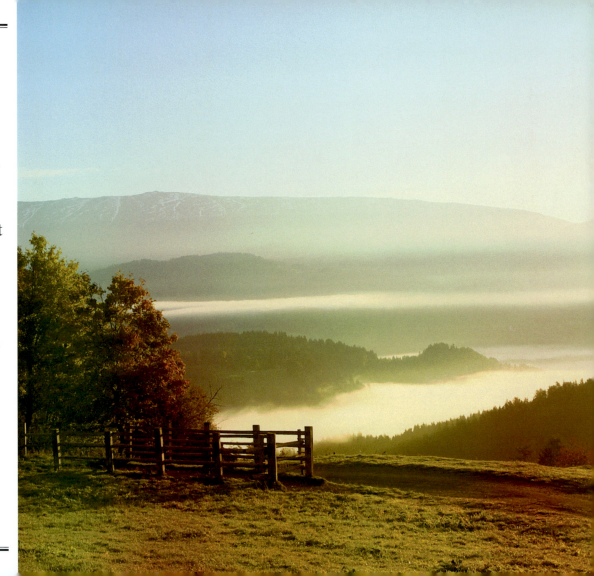

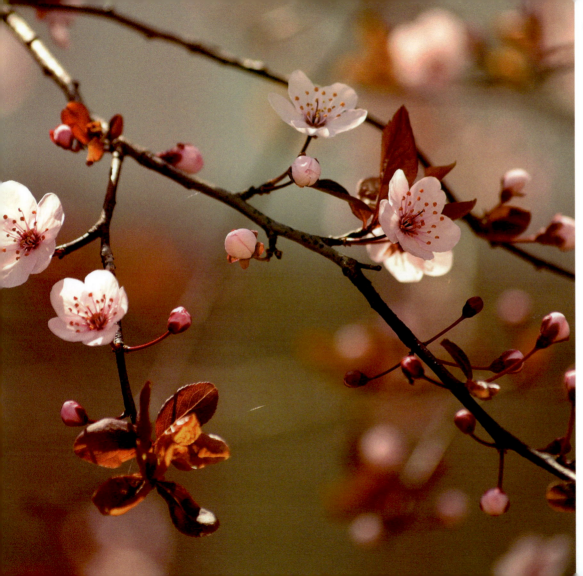

Refresh, Renew, Improve

I place *Forgiveness* over the top of my head and I allow myself to create a space where I can see the beauty inside me.

I take control of my past, move forward in strength and consider a better future.

I lovingly and willingly release and allow my body to be open to new possibilities for realizing my highest potential.

I rub *Gratitude* over my heart and forehead and I allow myself to see my true identity.

I am grateful for the peace that fills my body and opens my heart up to love.

I feel peace and love fill my body, mind and soul which relaxes me to create a life of emotional freedom.

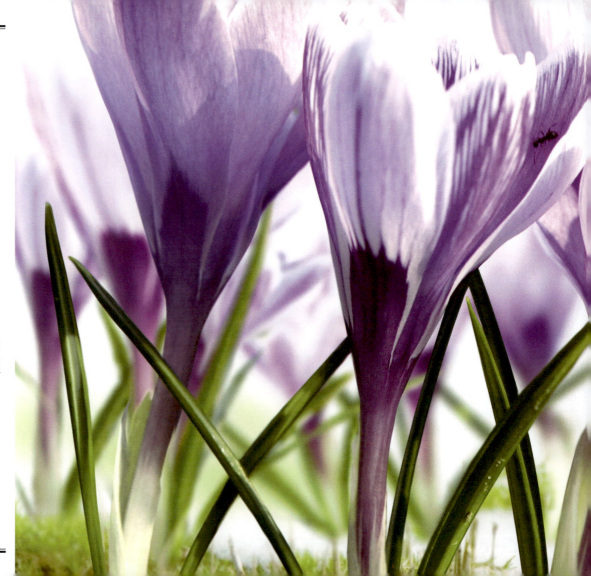

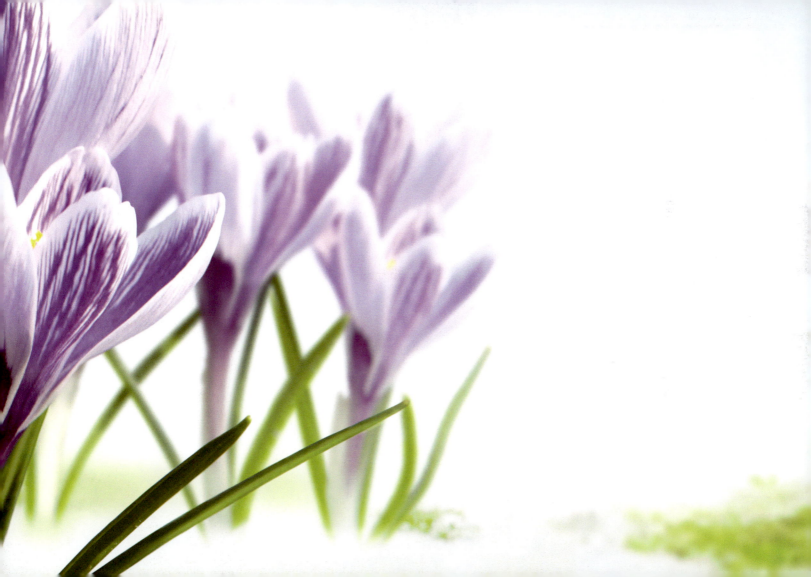

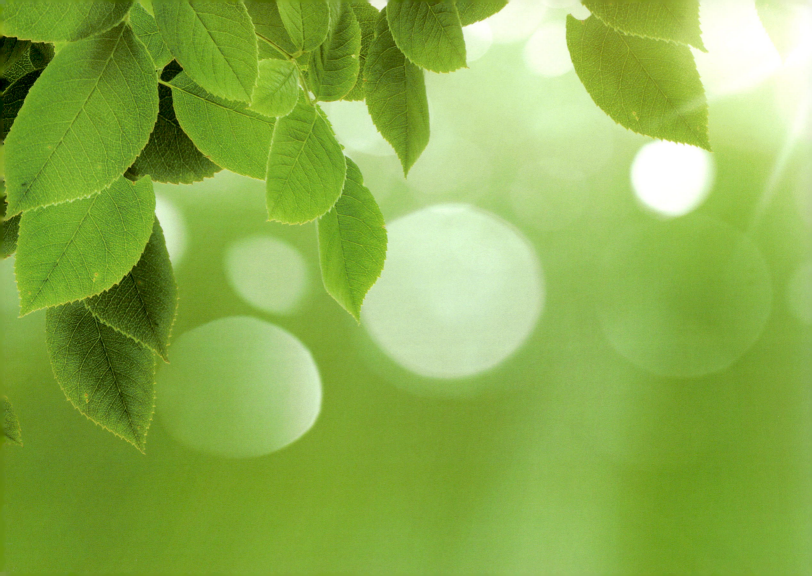

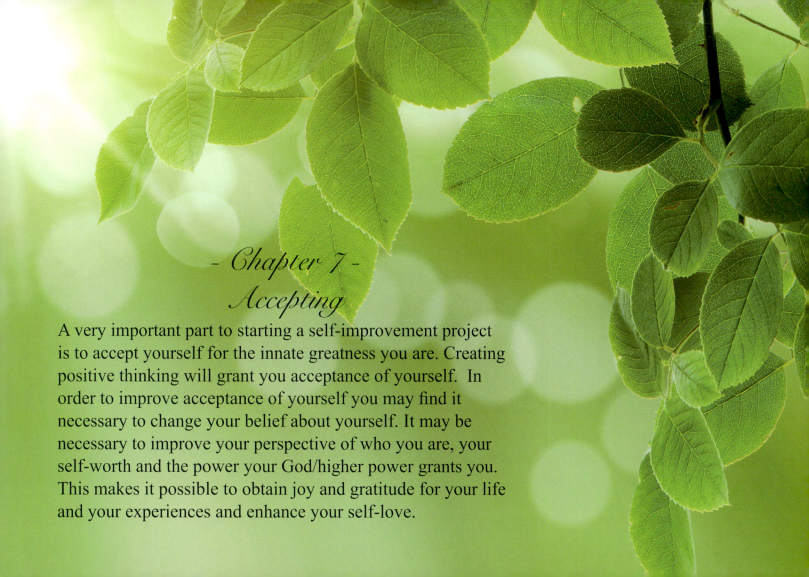

- Chapter 7 -
Accepting

A very important part to starting a self-improvement project is to accept yourself for the innate greatness you are. Creating positive thinking will grant you acceptance of yourself. In order to improve acceptance of yourself you may find it necessary to change your belief about yourself. It may be necessary to improve your perspective of who you are, your self-worth and the power your God/higher power grants you. This makes it possible to obtain joy and gratitude for your life and your experiences and enhance your self-love.

I brush *Inner Child* over my navel and connect with myself and draw upon my strengths.

I see my true identity, connect with my space of emotional freedom and accept myself for the greatness I am.

I allow my inner-child to acknowledge the power I possess to realize my highest potential.

I allow my inner-child to feel loved and accepted.

I allow my God/higher power to communicate with my inner-self and build a stronger me.

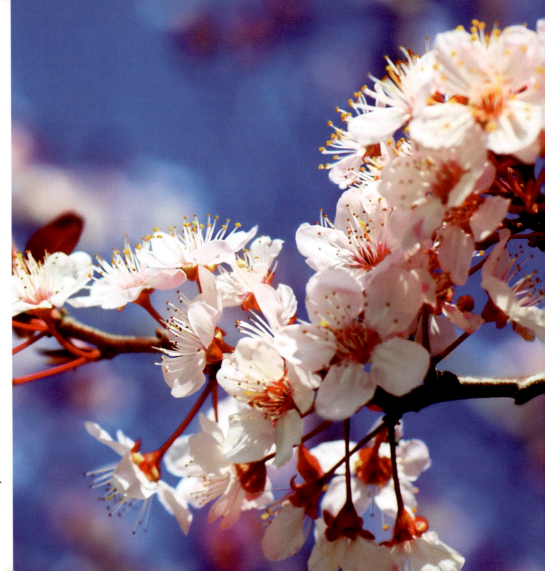

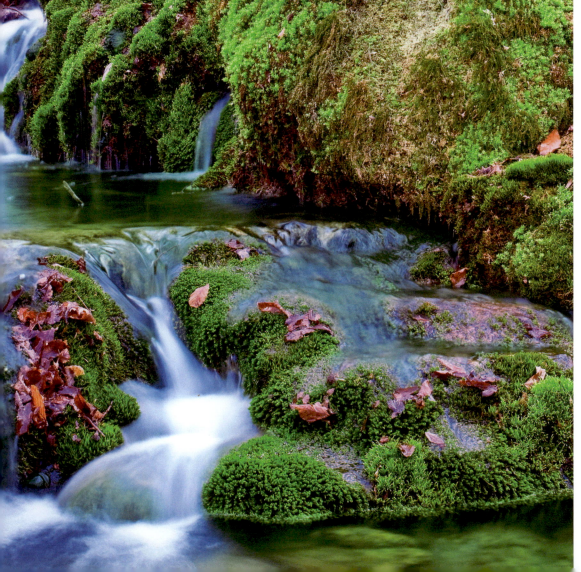

Refresh, Renew, Improve

I place *Release* over my liver and I allow myself to acknowledge and feel strength from within me build.

I allow my body to accept an inner peace and beauty.

I allow myself to acknowledge I am safe in the here-and-now.

I see a fresh me to shine forward and thank myself for positive changes I create.

I apply *Clarity* to the top of my head and allow myself to clearly develop and acknowledge a life I love.

I clearly allow my mind to open up to encouraging and uplifting thoughts that grant acceptance of myself.

I inhale the beautiful aroma and feel my emotional balance increase.

I clearly see joy and love for myself.

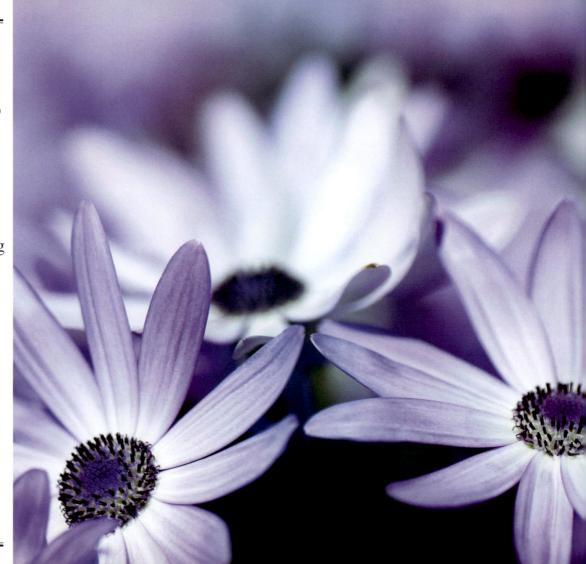

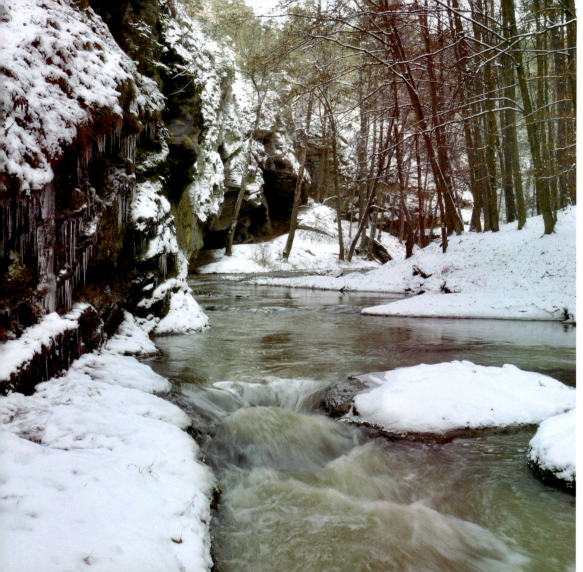

Refresh, Renew, Improve

I hold the bottle of *Dream Catcher* in my hand at night and feel safety as I sleep and relax.

I encourage and enhance my mental well-being and love who I am.

I realize I can please myself and accept me.

I place *Envision* over my third eye to feel and see the beauty inside myself.

I experience my life the way I envision it to be.

I create for myself balance and allow uplifting thoughts to surround my body, mind and soul.

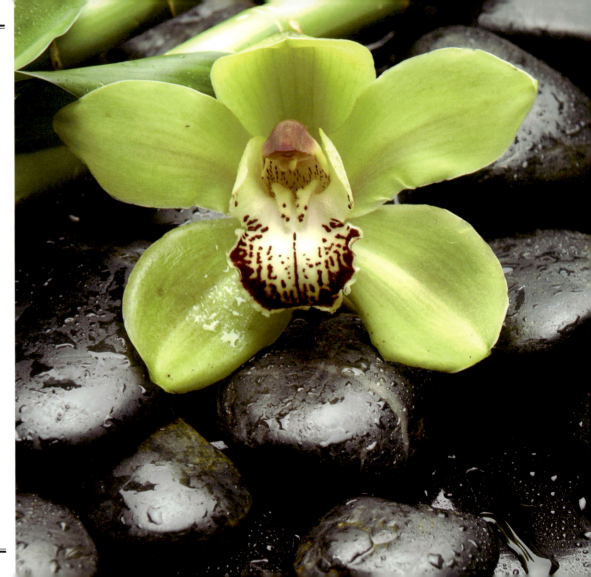

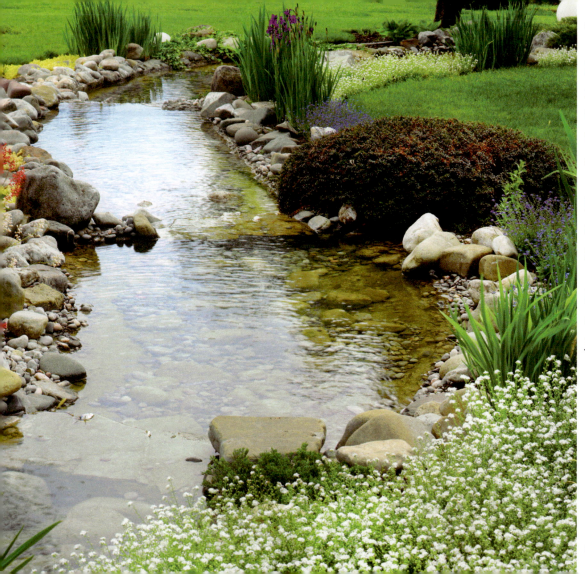

Refresh, Renew, Improve

I place *Into-the-Future* on my forehead and I accept the support necessary to move forward with comfort and ease.

I acknowledge self-improvement where I generate positive thoughts.

I recognize I love myself and choose to enjoy my journey.

I apply *Evergreen Essence* to my heart and I allow my body to have peace that surrounds me.

I control my thoughts and allow healing to uplift my body, mind and soul.

I allow my body to create an acceptable life for me to realize my life's purpose.

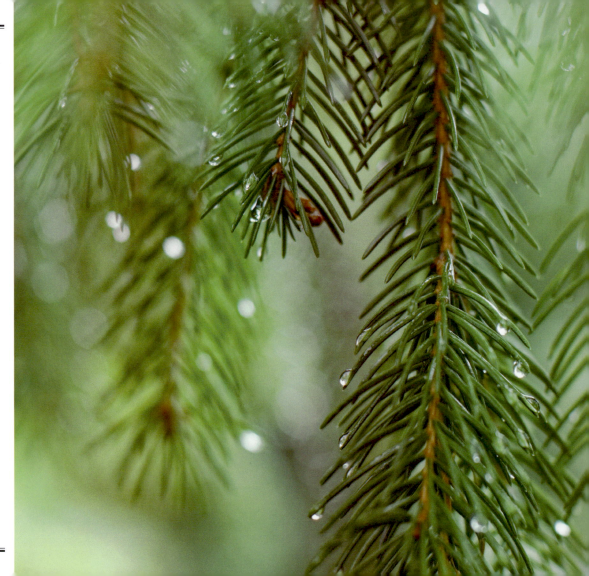

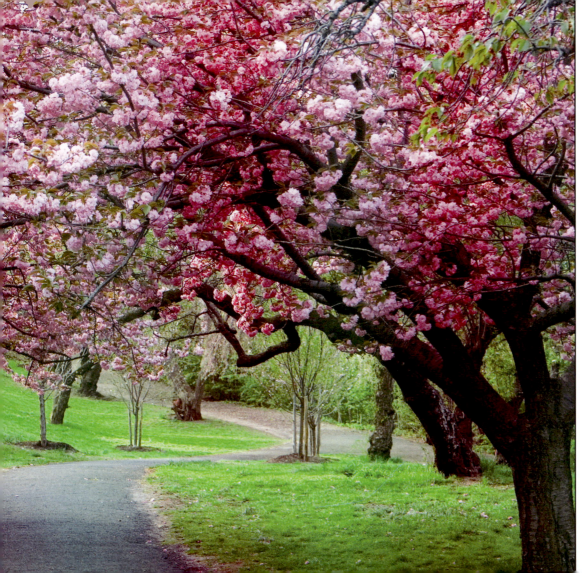

Refresh, Renew, Improve

I rub *Gathering* across my forehead and I allow my emotions to be centered and balanced.

I accept white light into my body, mind and soul and allow it to assist me in realizing my highest potential.

I move into a new light full of uplifting and soothing acceptance of me for the greatness I am.

I apply *Grounding* to my feet and I feel strength as my body, mind and soul are anchored in emotional stability.

I am grounded in who I am, in my great worth, and love for myself.

I am anchored in the here-and-now and feel at peace with my body, mind and soul.

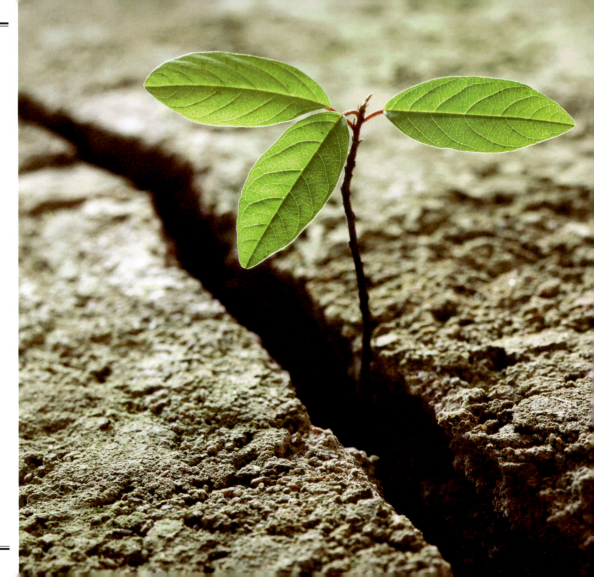

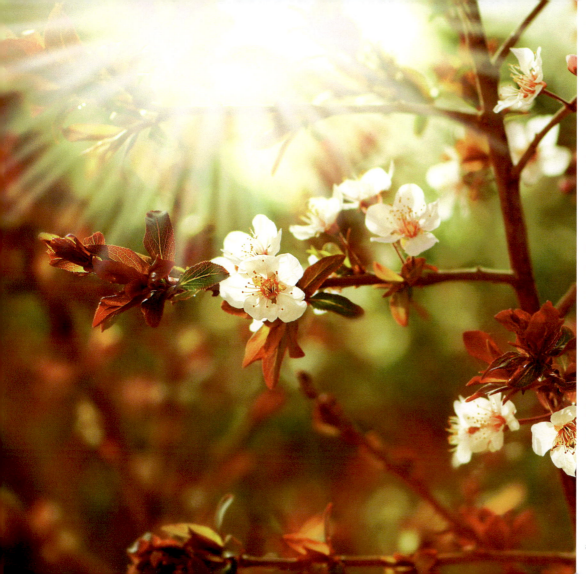

Refresh, Renew, Improve

I rub *Gratitude* over my heart and I feel grateful for all my God/higher power gives me that allows me to accept my divine worth.

I am grateful my life is balanced and I love my body for what it does for me each day.

I am grateful I accept emotional freedom and I gain a spiritual perspective of my life's purpose.

I am grateful for the many souls who touched my life as I touch theirs.

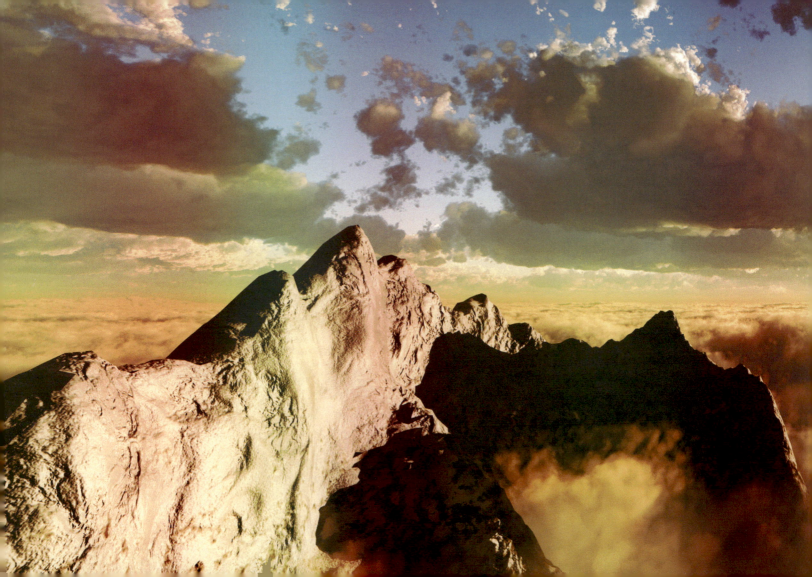

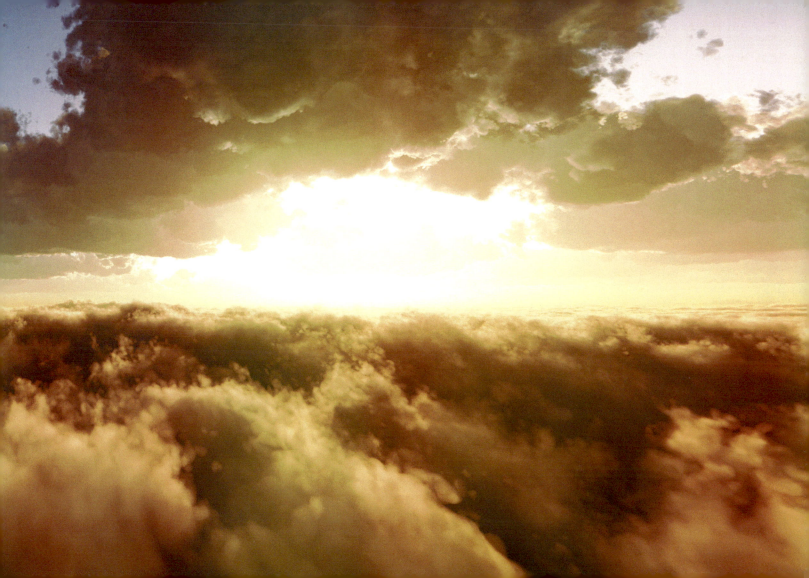

Notes

Notes

Notes